PSYCHIATRIC MONOGRAPH SERIES: 3

A TREATISE ON MADNESS
By William Battie, M.D.

AND

REMARKS ON DR. BATTIE'S TREATISE ON MADNESS
By John Monro, M.D.

PSYCHIATRIC MONOGRAPH SERIES

1. *Daniel Paul Schreber: memoirs of my nervous illness.* Translated and edited, with notes, introduction and discussion by Ida Macalpine and Richard Hunter, 1955.

2. *Schizophrenia 1677: a psychiatric study of an illustrated autobiographical record of demoniacal possession.* By Ida Macalpine and Richard Hunter, 1956.

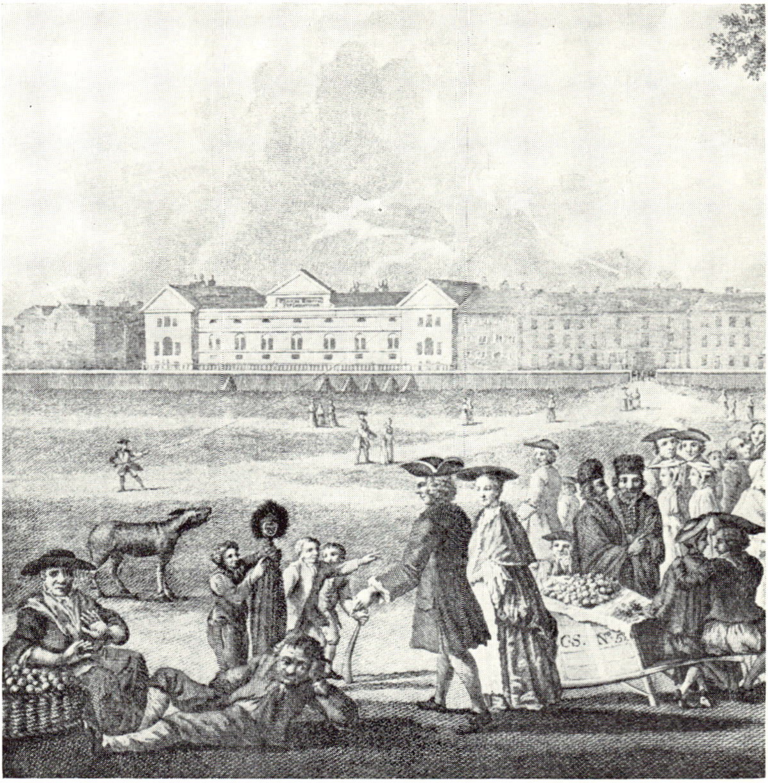

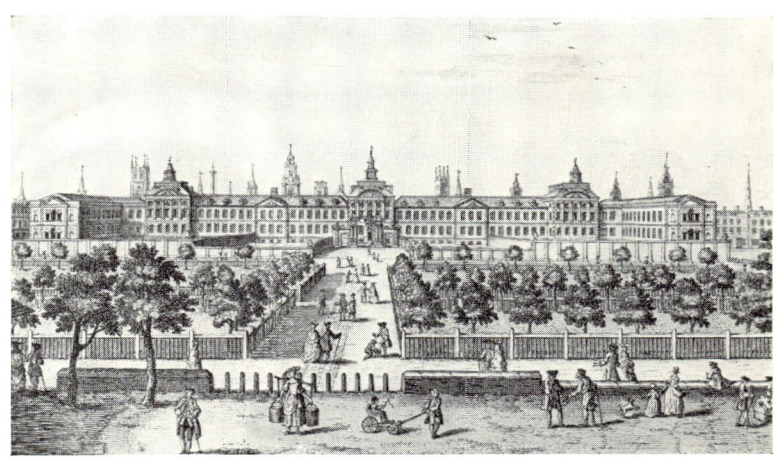

The first St. Luke's Hospital on Windmill Hill, London

Bethlem Hospital, *post* 1736

A Treatise on Madness

BY WILLIAM BATTIE, M.D.

AND

Remarks on Dr. Battie's Treatise on Madness

BY JOHN MONRO, M.D.

A Psychiatric Controversy of the Eighteenth Century

INTRODUCED AND ANNOTATED BY

RICHARD HUNTER
M.D., M.R.C.P., D.P.M.

AND

IDA MACALPINE
M.D., M.R.C.P.

1962
DAWSONS OF PALL MALL
LONDON

Published by
Dawsons of Pall Mall
16 Pall Mall
London, S.W.1

Introduction © Wm. Dawson & Sons Ltd, 1962
Printed in Great Britain by
The Hollen Street Press Ltd.
London W.1

CONTENTS

Introduction by Richard Hunter and Ida Macalpine
Notes
A Treatise on Madness by William Battie, M.D.
Remarks on Dr. Battie's Treatise on Madness
by John Monro, M.D.

ILLUSTRATIONS

Frontispiece. The first St. Luke's Hospital on Windmill Hill, London. (*Top*)
Bethlem Hospital, *post* 1736. (*Bottom*)

Fig. 1. Part of a print by William Hogarth (1735) depicting a madhouse. *Page* 8.

Fig. 2. Record of patients admitted and discharged at St. Luke's Hospital, 1751-65. *Page* 12.

ACKNOWLEDGEMENTS

The editors thank the Trustees of the British Museum; the Governors of King Edward's School, Witley (keepers of the old Bethlem records); the Trustees of the Methodist Church, London; the Registrar of the Royal College of Physicians, London; the Governors of St. Luke's-Woodside Hospital; and the President and Council of the Royal College of Surgeons of England for permission to quote from manuscript material.

INTRODUCTION

THE re-issue of Battie's *Treatise* and Monro's *Remarks* both published in 1758 allows the modern reader not only to participate in a celebrated psychiatric controversy and meet two leading physicians of the time, but also to gain a picture of psychiatry at a turning point in its history.

BETHLEM HOSPITAL

Until the middle of the eighteenth century the history of the insane had been almost coeval with the history of Bethlem Hospital, originally a priory belonging to the Order of St. Mary of Bethlehem where shelter was given to poor lunatics as early as the end of the fourteenth century. A hundred and fifty years later in 1547 when Henry VIII dissolved the monastries he presented it to the city of London as a hospital for poor lunatics. It remained the only hospital of its kind in the country until 1751, not counting three early eighteenth century foundations of little significance, Bethel Hospital, Norwich, opened 1724 and in London the 'lunatic wards' for the chronic insane at Guy's 1728 and at the French Protestant Hospital 1737. So ancient and entrenched in the popular mind was Bethlem's monopoly that 'bedlam' was synonymous with madness, madmen and madhouses.

From 1676 to 1816 Bethlem occupied the building in Moorfields with the incongruously majestic frontage designed by Robert Hooke and the famous statues of mania and melancholy by C. G. Cibber over its portal; wings for male and female 'incurables' were added in the 1730s when it housed about two hundred and fifty patients (see Frontispiece). Although physicians had been appointed to the Hospital since the end of the sixteenth century (some of whom like Edward Tyson were distinguished in other fields) none had written on the subject or their patients, nor made any advance on the centuries' old methods of treatment. Patients were kept chained in straw, and bled, purged and vomited at set seasons, and their diet was spare in accordance with the antiphlogistic or 'depleting system'

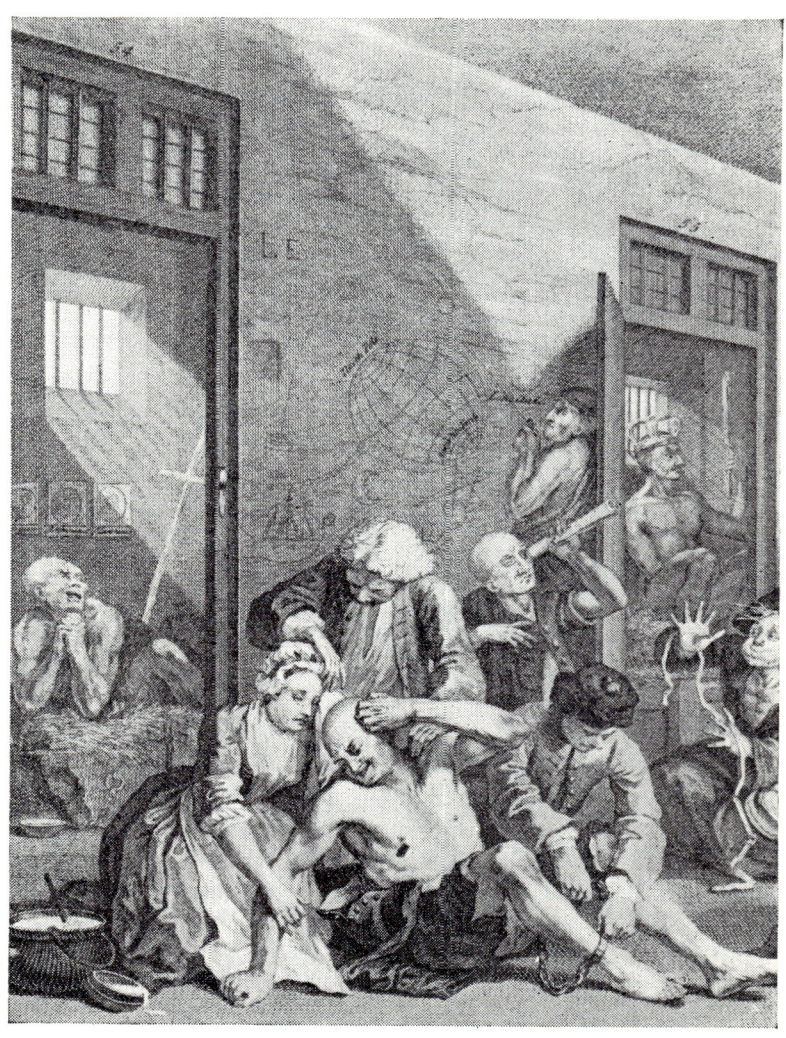

Fig. 1. Part of a print by William Hogarth (1735) depicting a madhouse

INTRODUCTION

designed to 'lower' turbulent spirits. Upon this scene of stagnation and unassailed tradition William Battie appeared and gave impetus and a fresh direction to the development of psychiatry.

WILLIAM BATTIE

He was born in 1703, the son of the vicar of Modbury in Devon, and educated at Eton and King's College, Cambridge on a Craven Scholarship in gratitude for which he later endowed the Battie Scholarship with a stipend of £20 annually. He gained repute as a classical scholar by his editions of Aristotle's *Rhetoric* (Cambridge 1728) and Isocrates's *Orations* (Cambridge 1729; second edition London 1749); and as demonstrator of anatomy had Horace Walpole among his pupils. In 1732 he obtained the licence *ad practicandum* and set up at Uxbridge, supported by his friends among them the Provost of Eton, Dr. Godolphin who to give him prestige in the neighbourhood sent his coach and four for the young doctor. In 1737 he took the M.D. and moved to London to a house in Great Russell Street next to Montague House, the future British Museum, where records show that as early as 1759 he was admitted to the Reading Room and allowed the use of the gardens with his family. His three daughters were celebrated by Gilbert White (brother of Benjamin White of the firm which published the *Treatise on madness*) in a poem 'To the Miss Batties', prefixed to the second edition of his *Natural history of Selborne*, 1813.

In 1738 he was elected Fellow of the Royal College of Physicians and established himself as a successful physician in the metropolis and a popular figure as a 'funster'. Stories of his puckish humour are recorded in John Nichol's *Literary anecdotes of the eighteenth century*, 1812, volume 4. In the College he soon achieved office, was Harveian Orator in 1746, and gave the Lumleian Lectures 1749-54 which were published in parts and as a collected edition *De principiis animalibus*, 1757. In 1760 appeared *Aphorismi de cognoscendis & curandis morbis*, a medical text based on physiological principles 'after the manner of Boerhaave'. Finally he rose to the highest medical honour when he was chosen President of the College in 1764. He had by then long devoted himself exclusively to the study and treatment of the insane and was – and remains to this day – the only psychiatrist to hold this office. That he achieved this professional eminence

INTRODUCTION

from the 'mad-business' as he called it, an unpromising if not actually disreputable and hence neglected field, brought it to the notice of other physicians and encouraged them to follow his lead and take it up. In the course of time this led to it acquiring social and professional respectability, a development accelerated by the widespread interest aroused by George III's illness in 1788 and the ignorance the Royal physicians had to admit when publicly examined by Parliamentary Committees on their knowledge and experience of insanity. The result was that by the turn of the century psychiatry was fairly established as an accepted medical specialty and regular physicians had taken the place of the quacks who had notoriously exploited the insane before.

In 1742 Battie was elected Fellow of the Royal Society. To the same year can be traced the first record of his interest in psychiatry, when by subscribing fifty guineas he had himself elected a governor of Bethlem Hospital, and from the old Committee Books the surprising fact emerges that for the rest of his life he took an active part in its affairs. Indeed in 1775, the year before he died, he was a candidate for the post of Treasurer, the most powerful executive of the Charity. He served on many Committees, among them those which set up the first 'apothecary's shop' or dispensary in the Hospital, 1751; which appointed John Monro as joint physician with his father James, 1751, and sole physician in succession, 1752; which abolished sightseeing in the Hospital at a penny or twopence a time, 1770; and which created the office of 'resident apothecary' or medical officer, 1772 (after the example of St. Luke's, 1766), a post which John Haslam filled 1795-1816.

ST. LUKE'S HOSPITAL

It seems that what Battie saw at Bethlem impressed him with the urgent need for a fresh approach and when he had gained sufficient practical experience in a private madhouse of his own, he began to canvass for the establishment of a second foundation for the poor and mad which was to create a new standard of care and treatment. He visualised that it should also provide the opportunity for students to observe patients as a first step to raising professional standards and status. It opened with Battie as its physician in July 1751 as St. Luke's Hospital for Lunaticks

INTRODUCTION

(see the Frontispiece) on the site known as the Foundry on Windmill Hill, on the north side of what today is Finsbury Square and what was then Moorfields, opposite Bethlem. John Wesley's Meeting House had been on the site since 1739 and when the Hospital took it over he became its tenant at a rental of £9 per annum, and, as the Committee Books record, attended several meetings. The founders explained in their Prospectus:

> The Principal End ... of establishing another Hospitall for *Lunaticks* is evident, not only as they are incapable of providing for themselves and Families, are not admitted into other Hospitalls, or capable of being relieved (as in other Diseases) by private Charity: but also as there must be Servants peculiarly qualified, and every Patient must have a separate Room, and Diet, most of them, equal to Persons in Health ... Although the only end hereby proposed was to establish a Charity ... Yet some Advantages of a very interesting Nature to the good of all Mankind, certainly will arise in Consequence of it; For more Gentlemen of the Faculty, making this Branch of Physick their particular Care and Study, it may from thence reasonably be expected that the Cure of this dreadful Disease will hereafter be rendered more certain and expeditious, as well as less expensive.

It was the first hospital in which attempts were made at a more rational approach to insanity, and where the insane were treated not by a routine of coercion and physicking but rather by 'regimen' and 'management'. This grew into the 'moral treatment' of the nineteenth century–the humanizing of the patient's life in the asylum, replacing medical control by self-control, idleness by work, and apathy by interest and occupation according to the needs of the case. Here in 1753 for the first time anywhere in the world students were permitted to walk the wards of an asylum and were given clinical instruction by Battie (the governors of Bethlem refused to admit students for another ninety years). Among his pupils who later rose to eminence was Sir George Baker, physician to George III.

Subsequent history shows that the new rival establishment long maintained its initial lead, and its record remained free from the scandals which marred the reputation of Bethlem in the next hundred years. Indeed when the cruelties and abuses which were discovered at Bethlem led to the historic Parliamentary inquiry into the state of madhouses, 1815-6, St. Luke's was held up as a well conducted institution. Before then its example

YEAR	ADMITTED Male	Fem.	Total	CURED Male	Fem.	Paralytic, Epileptic, Idiotic, and unfit from Disease. Male	Fem.	By desire of Friends. Male	Fem.	Proving to be with Child.	Proving not to be Lunatic. Fem.	Friends not complying with the Rules. Male	Fem.	Not being objects of Charity. Male	Fem.	Having been discharged uncured from Bethlem. Male	Fem.	Having been Insane above twelve months. Male	Fem.	Dead. Male	Fem.	Uncured, having been twelve months in Hospital. Male	Fem.	REMAINING at the end of the respective Years. Male	Fem.	Total
1751	10	33	43	3	6	2	4	...	...	...	...	...	...	...	...	...	...	...	...	1	2	...	...	4	21	25
1752	19	56	75	5	24	4	9	...	1	1	...	...	...	...	...	...	...	...	...	1	...	...	9	13	33	46
1753	20	51	71	7	26	2	1	1	5	...	...	...	...	...	...	...	...	...	...	1	1	6	16	15	35	50
1754	21	52	73	6	32	3	3	1	1	...	...	1	1	1	...	...	...	...	...	2	2	8	13	14	35	49
1755	20	53	73	10	20	1	1	...	7	...	...	1	...	...	...	...	...	...	...	2	4	7	20	14	36	50
1756	28	42	70	8	29	4	2	2	2	...	...	...	1	...	...	...	...	...	...	2	2	5	18	21	25	46
1757	21	58	79	19	25	4	3	...	1	...	...	...	1	...	...	...	...	...	...	2	2	7	14	9	38	47
1758	24	64	88	15	28	2	4	1	2	...	...	...	...	1	...	...	...	...	...	...	3	6	24	9	40	49
1759	32	47	79	9	33	5	3	1	2	...	...	...	...	...	...	...	...	...	...	4	2	3	17	18	30	48
1760	30	54	84	18	26	3	3	...	1	...	...	...	...	1	...	...	1	...	...	1	6	8	18	18	30	48
1761	26	57	83	14	30	5	7	2	4	...	...	...	...	1	1	...	...	...	...	...	2	8	9	14	34	48
1762	28	52	80	11	28	2	8	...	2	...	1	...	...	...	...	...	1	...	...	2	2	7	14	20	30	50
1763	25	53	78	12	17	3	2	3	3	1	...	...	...	...	...	...	...	...	...	...	6	14	19	13	33	46
17F4	33	69	102	16	26	3	3	1	1	1	...	...	...	...	...	...	...	...	...	2	4	6	18	18	49	67
1765	33	73	106	8	32	6	7	2	1	1	...	...	...	...	...	...	...	...	...	4	5	10	30	21	46	67
Cd. ford.	370	814	1184	161	382	49	60	14	33	4	1	3	2	2	2	1	2	...	2	24	43	95	239	21	46	67

Fig. 2. Record of patients admitted and discharged at St. Luke's Hospital 1751-65.
From St. Luke's Centenary Report, 1851.

INTRODUCTION

had encouraged the founding of a number of provincial lunatic hospitals of which Manchester, 1766 was the first, followed by St. Luke's Newcastle-upon-Tyne, York, Liverpool and Leicester. In 1786 the Hospital moved to the gaunt premises on Old Street which Dickens visited in 1852 and described in *A curious dance round a curious tree*; in 1916 this building was taken over by the Bank of England as a printing works, and at the time of writing is awaiting demolition, while the Foundation continues as part of the Middlesex Hospital.

In 1764 at the age of sixty Battie retired from active work at the Hospital but remained to advise as a governor until his death in 1776. One thousand patients–more than one half of whom were discharged 'cured'–had been in his care. Christopher Smart was one of them (he was never a patient at Bethlem as is sometimes claimed) but was discharged uncured in May 1758 on Battie's report to his Weekly Committee that he 'continues disordered in his Senses notwithstanding he has been admitted into this Hospital above 12 Calender Months, and from the present Circumstances of his Case there not being sufficient reason to expect his speedy recovery'. This was the standard formula by which uncured patients were discharged, and, as at Bethlem, they could be readmitted on the incurable list.

BATTIE'S TREATISE

In December 1757 appeared the *Treatise on madness* dated 1758. From Elizabethan times there had been books on particular aspects of mental illness starting with Timothy Bright's *Treatise of melancholy*, 1586, followed by Edward Jorden's *Briefe discourse of a disease called the suffocation of the mother*, 1603 which introduced the concept of hysteria to English readers, and Robert Burton's encyclopedic *Anatomy of melancholy*, 1621. Nearer Battie's time, Sir Richard Blackmore (1725) and Nicholas Robinson (1729) had written on 'the spleen and vapours', Malcolm Flemyng had published his *Neuropathia* (1740) in Latin verse, and the mysterious P. Frings had issued his *Treatise on phrensy* (1746). But Battie's was the first 'on madness' and so entitled, and the first written from a large clinical experience by a practising specialist with a distinguished scientific and professional background. Most important it was written in conformity with the intention of the founders of St. Luke's, of 'introducing

INTRODUCTION

more Gentlemen of the Faculty to the Study and Practice of one of the most important branches of Physick', for those 'Students, who have not the same opportunity of seeing practice'.

Although entitled *A treatise* it was in no sense a textbook but rather an essay intended to open up a field which had lain fallow and obscured by old attitudes, classifications and treatments. Battie pointed out that the variety of terms in use showed the primitive state of the subject, and criticised the fanciful speculations about the functions of the brain and nerves on which theories and therapies were based – a theme he had discussed at length in his Lumleian Lectures. He himself was abreast of 'recent advances' in physiology, as for instance Albrecht von Haller's distinction of nervous irritability from muscular contractility which he was the first to propound in this country. Taking his cue from the physiology of sensation, he defined madness as 'deluded imagination', a view contrary to the one then generally held that it was a manifestation of 'vitiated judgment' needing correction by violent treatments and coercive measures. This at least opened the door to interest in the problems of the individual patient, and certainly paved the way for milder treatment which Battie strongly advocated. A physician in the Hippocratic tradition, he respected the processes of nature and their power to heal in mind as much as in body, and was shocked by the shocking therapies in use, although he realised it was 'almost haeretical to impeach their antimaniacal virtues'. He scorned as remnants of the dark ages the empirics who knew nothing of the diseases they so assiduously combated with their 'solemn parade of medicaments' – the approach to practice epitomised by that arch therapist Everard Maynwaring who held it 'much more necessary, that the Physitian look into the medicine then the chamber-pot' (*Tutela sanitatis*, 1664). In his Harveian Oration devoted to the same theme, he took as his exemplars the great physicians of the past: Thomas Sydenham for instance, who fought the *furor therapeuticus* of his time and brought the spirit of scientific observation into medical practice. Almost one hundred years after him Battie introduced the same rational spirit of expectant observation to psychiatry and reiterated its first principle, that 'we should take great care not to do harm where it is not in our power to do any good'.

INTRODUCTION

Not only did he consider some of the methods of treatment reprehensible, but, he pointed out, their application to all cases of 'Madness' alike implied that it was 'one species of disorder', whereas 'when thoroughly examined, it discovers as much variety with respect to its causes and circumstances as any distemper whatever. Madness therefore . . . rejects all general methods'. He proposed as a working classification a simple division into 'Original' and 'Consequential' madness, the one without, the other consequent upon brain disease. This differentiation of the non-organic – the group of mental illnesses proper – from the organic – the mental manifestations of cerebral disease – was a fundamental advance and the boldness of Battie's conception is the more striking when it is remembered that neuropathology was not much advanced beyond what Thomas Willis had observed on the 'brain and nervous stock' in the previous century (*Pathologiae cerebri, et nervosi generis specimen*, 1667; *De anima brutorum*, 1672).

Battie blamed chiefly the physicians of Bethlem for this state of affairs in which a host of false facts, false theories and irrational treatments had been allowed to continue to obscure fundamental ignorance and so obstruct progress. 'The difficulties attending the care of Lunaticks have been at least perpetuated by their being entrusted to Empiricks' he wrote, 'or at best to a few select Physicians, most of whom thought it adviseable to keep the cases as well as the patients to themselves'. This reference was made still more pointed in the annual *Reasons for the establishing and further encouragement of St. Luke's Hospital for Lunaticks*, which contained the report of the year's cases, the Hospital's rules, a list of subscribers, etc. where it was bluntly stated that the subject had been 'already too long confined (almost) to a single Person'.

MONRO'S REMARKS

Four months later the physician of Bethlem, John Monro, published his vindication, *Remarks on Dr. Battie's treatise*. Of the two books it is today much the rarer perhaps because as its inferior production indicates, it was not meant to stand by itself. Even so it has the distinction of being the first contribution to psychiatry to come from Bethlem Hospital, and it is to Battie's credit to have provoked it. 'My own inclination would never have led me

INTRODUCTION

to appear in print' exclaimed Monro, 'but it was thought necessary for me, in my situation, to say something in answer to the undeserved censures, which Dr. Battie has thrown upon my predecessors'. Speaking for himself he confessed 'Madness is a distemper of such a nature, that very little of real use can be said concerning it'; as to the earlier physicians of Bethlem and more particularly his father, 'Though they did not publish their thoughts on a distemper which was more immediately the object of their care, that was not owing to any design of keeping their manner of practice a secret, but that they thought it disingenuous, to perplex mankind, with points that must for ever remain dark, intricate, and uncertain'. However, finding himself forced if only by filial piety to make this public reply, he confined himself to a satirical and at times scathing commentary on the *Treatise*, section by section, the tenor of which was declared by the Horatian motto on the title-page: 'O greater madman, pray have mercy on a lesser one'.

But just as Battie had set himself against the traditional system to which Monro was heir, so Monro fought on medical issues, not personal grounds, and ridiculed the new doctrine, not its author. Battie's three major innovations came in for his severest strictures: 'I should rather define madness to be vitiated judgment' he wrote, and 'of what value it may hereafter prove to have thus divided madness into original and consequential is not my business to enquire at present. The first of these is entirely the doctor's invention it never having been mentioned by any writer, or observed by any physician. . . . The manner indeed of ranging madness under several causes is new, but will not, I fear, be of any great use'. Of treatment 'I will venture to say, that the most adequate and constant cure of it is by evacuation' and of these 'vomiting is infinitely preferable to any other' next to 'bleeding and purging' and 'issues between the shoulders'. 'Why' he remonstrated, 'should we endeavour to give the world a shocking opinion of a remedy, that is not only safe, but greatly useful . . . I should be very sorry to find anyone frightened from the use of such an efficacious remedy by it's being called a shocking operation, the consequence of a morbid convulsion'.

Having countered Battie's every point, Monro at the conclusion of his book left it 'to the impartiality of the publick to determine between the *Treatise* and the *Remarks*' and modestly added

INTRODUCTION

'If Dr. Battie has miscarried in his undertaking, I cannot think that the judicious reader will be HEREBY inclined to turn his thoughts to the same subject'.

If by 'judicious reader' Monro meant the general public, they very soon did turn their attention to madness and madhouses, to lunatics and their keepers; if he meant the profession, they too were forced from then on to acknowledge psychiatry. The fillip it gained resulted not only from the publicity of this controversy, but also because it revealed that there existed a sufficient body of experience for experts to disagree.

'Both the *Treatise* and the *Remarks* are the works of men very eminent in their profession, especially in that branch on which they treat' wrote Tobias Smollett in *The Critical Review*, March 1758. 'If Dr. Battie has reflected on the late Dr. [James] Monro, the son has vindicated him with spirit. . . . They are rivals in fame, and hitherto the contest is conducted with spirit and decorum, free from personal abuse, and abounding with matter of real utility . . . and as such [we] recommend it to our ingenious and medical readers'. Smollett himself apparently found some passages so entertaining that he plagiarised them in his novel *Sir Launcelot Greaves*, 1762. James Boswell when writing on hypochondriasis quoted Battie's *Treatise*–'a book sufficiently corporeal'–and mentions having visited the incurables at St. Luke's 'out of sad curiosity' (*The hypochondriack*, 1782, no. 63).

More important the impetus they gave to psychiatry is reflected in the crop of psychiatric books which followed later in the century, all of which are indebted to Battie and Monro. As late as 1810 when Dr. Matthew Baillie was called to George III in his last attack of insanity and wanted information on it, he wrote to his wife from Windsor 'be so good as to procure for me Dr. Battie's Treatise . . . and the old Dr. Monro's remarks upon that treatise'.

JAMES MONRO

John Monro was of the second generation of the remarkable Monro family, four generations of which provided physicians to Bethlem Hospital in uninterrupted succession for one hundred and twenty five years, from 1728 to 1853; in the fifth generation Henry Monro (1817-1891), the last psychiatrist of the line, by a curious quirk of fate became physician to St. Luke's Hospital in

INTRODUCTION

1855 and incidentally was the only member of the family who contributed spontaneously to the advancement of psychiatry and indeed neurology by his writings. They were descended from the Reverend Alexander Monro of Fyrish, Principal of Edinburgh University, who was dispossessed after the Revolution and came to London in 1690. His second son James (1680-1752) M.D. Oxon, F.R.C.P. was a general physician before he was appointed to Bethlem in 1728. The first mad-doctor of the dynasty, his name became associated with all matters lunatic to an extent none of his predecessors or successors ever achieved; so much so that even Battie in his earlier days was referred to as 'the Monro of his time'. This renown came his way not by virtue of any contribution to the specialty—he told his friend Sir Robert Walpole, the Prime Minister, that 'he scarce knew anything that asses' milk and change of air would not cure'—nor simply because he was the only doctor in and around London for such cases. He owed it chiefly to the growth of periodical literature at that time, and through the columns of the press his name became a household word. In *The Gentleman's Magazine* (founded in 1731) for instance, a correspondent wrote in May 1739: 'I hope we are not so far gone in Madness or corruption, as to think that the Nation and the People were made for the Use of the Persons at the Helm. If so, Doctor *Monro* is the only Minister that can help us'. Alexander Pope in whose circle Monro moved, also has many references to him and his Hospital as in the following lines from *The dunciad*:

> Close to those walls where Folly holds her throne,
> And laughs to think Monro would take her down.

Glimpses into his practice may be gained from contemporary accounts, the most detailed of which is Alexander Cruden's who broke down in 1738 after completing his *Concordance* and was treated by the 'Bethlemetical Doctor' in Wright's Madhouse at Bethnal Green. Whenever he came 'Monro, like a bird upon the wing, made only a standing visit' without giving him the chance to talk, and indeed prescribed vomits, purges, the lancet and had him straitwaistcoated and chained 'a week before he had visited him', as Cruden complained in *The London-Citizen exceedingly injured*, 1739. Incidentally, fifteen years later when he fell ill again, he was treated by John Monro in Duffield's Madhouse

INTRODUCTION

at Little Chelsea, an episode recounted in *The adventures of Alexander the Corrector*, 1754. On this occasion he just managed to escape coming under Battie's care by sleeping away from 'his lodgings the night betwixt Thursday and Friday, the time of seizing patients for *St. Luke's*' where he was on the waiting list. Susannah Wesley wrote to her son John, who had many contacts with the Monros, of 'that wretched Fellow Monro' who physicked patients who had 'much more need of a Spiritual, than Bodily Physician'.

JOHN MONRO

James Monro's son John (1715-1791) was born at Greenwich and educated at Merchant Taylors' School and St. John's College, Oxford where he graduated M.A. in 1740. The following year he was elected to a Radcliffe Travelling Fellowship and studied medicine at Edinburgh, Leyden and in France, Germany and Italy. In 1747 he became M.D. Oxon, in 1748 a governor of Bethlem Hospital, and in 1751 joint physician and in 1752 sole physician in succession to his father. In 1753 he was elected Fellow of the Royal College of Physicians and was on several occasions Censor. His tastes were classical and his gifts artistic, he was a Fellow of the Society of Antiquaries and of the Royal Society of Arts, and assembled a fine library and collection of engravings which were sold after his death by Leigh & Sotheby, 1792. His private madhouse, Brooke House, Hackney, a historic building destroyed by bombing in 1940, is the subject of a monograph in the London County Council Series *Survey of London*, 1960. He gave expression to his love of books in his Harveian Oration, 1757 by lauding the British Museum as 'a noble and worthy undertaking' which 'though scarcely begun, surpasses the most celebrated libraries in Europe'. He himself was a fair draughtsman as surviving drawings show, a family gift which became more pronounced in later generations. His son and successor Thomas (1758-1833)–who like all the Monros of Bethlem left psychiatry as he found it–was a distinguished water colourist, connoisseur and patron of the arts, famous as the founder of the British school of watercolourists who counted Turner and Girtin among his protégés. Thomas's grandson Henry, who has already been mentioned, was a gifted painter whose family portraits hang in the Royal College of Physicians.

INTRODUCTION

The long years of service given to the insane by the Monros are clouded by the fact that both Thomas in 1816 and his son and successor Edward Thomas (1790-1856) in 1853 were dismissed from their posts at Bethlem as the result of the public enquiries of 1815-6 and 1852 which revealed malpractices at the Hospital for which they were held responsible.

BATTIE AND MONRO

It would be a mistake to assume that relations between the two men were strained by their differences of opinion. Pamphleteering was an accepted eighteenth century method of putting forward contrary views even among friends, and all the evidence points to Battie and Monro having continued harmonious relations. They met frequently at the College and worked together at Bethlem, the one as governor, the other as physician. When a Parliamentary Committee sat in 1763 to enquire into 'The Manner of admitting Persons into Houses now kept for the Reception of Lunatics; And, The Treatment of them during their Confinement' both Battie and Monro gave evidence to the same effect and nearly in the same words, namely 'That private Madhouses require some better Regulation ... that the Admission of Persons brought as Lunatic is too loose and too much at large ... and that frequent Visitation is necessary for the Inspection of the Lodging, Diet, Cleanliness, and Treatment'. Nine years earlier in 1754 the College had been approached by Sir Cordell Firebrass for the House of Commons, to ascertain whether they would be willing to supervise the madhouses of London. Monro was Censor at the time and Battie chosen to answer for the College that 'they apprehend the Execution of that Trust will be attended with such difficulties as will make it very inconvenient to the College to perform it'. Eventually the College did co-operate and in 1774 the first Act 'to regulate mad-houses' was passed which introduced medical certificates for patients admitted, and licensing and inspection of private asylums; in London the overseeing body became the College through five Fellows duly appointed Commissioners. The very first licence was taken out by Battie for his madhouse in Wood's Close, Clerkenwell and the second by Monro for Brooke House.

Battie and Monro also consulted together on many occasions.

INTRODUCTION

The best known of these occurred in 1763 when a former patient of Monro named Wood brought an action against him for falsely and maliciously detaining him 'as a lunatic'. Lord Mansfield who tried the case, many years later told Lord Erskine that Wood underwent the most rigorous examination by Monro's counsel without revealing a trace of mental illness, but when Battie was called he quickly made the patient unfold his delusional system and so saved the day for his colleague. This story became historic: Erskine quoted it at the trial of James Hadfield in 1800 for attempting the life of George III. It has been quoted ever since in medico-legal texts to show that insanity may not only not be obvious, but actually be concealed successfully, and detected only by expert psychiatric interviewing, as by Battie in Wood's case.

Monro's name is associated with two other famous criminal cases. In 1760 he was called as an expert witness at the trial of Earl Ferrers for the murder of his steward. Under cross examination he deposed that the commonest 'symptoms of lunacy' were 'uncommon fury . . . violence against other persons or against themselves . . . jealousy, or suspicion without cause' and occasionally 'the carrying of arms'. In 1786 with his son Thomas he examined Margaret Nicholson, who also attempted the life of the King, at the request of the Privy Council and declared her insane. Like Hadfield she was sent to Bethlem, but without being brought to trial. Monro's last appearance on the public scene was in 1788 when he was summoned to George III at the beginning of his first attack of insanity. He prescribed a pillow stuffed with hops for the Royal insomnia and was not called again on the grounds of age.

So ended a formative era in psychiatry and the supremacy of London. For the next decades the centre of progress shifted to the provinces, to Ferriar of Manchester, Perfect of West Malling, Arnold of Leicester, Pargeter of Reading, Cox of Bristol, and the lay Tuke family of York–to mention only some. It had begun with the controversy between Battie and Monro, those two colourful figures on the eighteenth century medical scene, the one *'faber fortunae suae'* and looking to the future, the other born into office and personifying the past.

NOTES ON BATTIE'S *TREATISE*

Page

28 'Mr. Locke': John Locke *An essay concerning humane understanding*, London, 1690, p. 126

32 'Willis': Thomas Willis *De anima brutorum*, London, 1672

32 'Stahl': Georg Ernst von Stahl *Theoria medica vera*, Halle, 1707

47 'Dover': Thomas Dover *The ancient physician's legacy to his country*, London, 1732

47 'Calenture': acute febrile delirium observed among sailors in the tropics

49 'Men prove with child . . .': Alexander Pope *The rape of the lock*, 1714, Canto IV, line 53

57 'meagrim': migraine, a corruption of hemicrania

64 'errhines': medicines taken as snuff to provoke nasal secretion and believed to purge the head and so clear the brain

68, last paragraph: a reference to the fact that Bethlem was still a public show despite almost a century of protests (*cf.* Thomas Tryon *A treatise of dreams and visions* [London, 1689], p. 290

75 'Dr. Mead': Richard Mead *Medical precepts and cautions*, translated from the Latin by T. Stack, London, 1751, p. 94

75 'sinapisms [mustard plasters], caustics and vesicatories': various forms of counter-irritant treatment

80 'alexipharmacs': remedies to expel poisons or the matter of disease by sweat (Robert James *A medicinal dictionary*, 3 vols, London, 1743-5)

91 'Extract. Thebaicum': also called Venetian treacle, a preparation of opium

95 'Anticyra': a town in Thessaly famed for its hellebore, the ancient remedy for madness

NOTES ON MONRO'S *REMARKS*

Page

1 'Aretæus': *The extant works of Aretæus*, edited and translated by F. Adams, London, 1856, p. 301 *ff.*

5 'Tully': Marcus Tullius Cicero

35 'the late physician of Bethlem': James Monro (1680-1752), John's father

47 'Celsus': A. Cornelius Celsus *Of medicine*, translated by James Greive, London, 1756, p. 147

50/1 'Treatment by evacuation': sixty years later the same treatments were still used at Bethlem as shown by the statement of Thomas Monro, John's son: 'They [the patients] are ordered to be bled about the latter end of May ... and after ... they take vomits once a week for a certain number of weeks, after that we purge the patients: that has been the practice invariably for years ... it was handed down to me by my father, and I do not know any better practice' (*First Report. Minutes of Evidence taken before the Select Committee appointed to consider of provision being made for the better regulation of madhouses, in England*, 1815, p. 95)

51 'Dr. Bryan Robinson': *Observations...*, London, 1752

52 'issues and setons': in later years Monro changed his mind about their usefulness and directed the surgeon at Bethlem to heal them (Bryan Crowther *Practical remarks on insanity*, London, 1811, pp. 42-3)

BIBLIOGRAPHICAL NOTE

A Treatise on madness by William Battie, M.D., was first published in 1758 in quarto (dimensions of the copy measured 10 x 7½ inches). In this lithographic reprint the text has been reproduced in facsimile but the size of the page has been reduced.

Remarks on Dr. Battie's treatise on madness by John Monro, M.D., was published in 1758 in octavo (dimensions of the copy measured 7¾ x 4¾ inches). In this reprint the width of the type panel has been photographically enlarged from 20 ems to 24½ ems pica.

A TREATISE ON MADNESS.

By WILLIAM BATTIE M. D.

Fellow of the College of Physicians in LONDON,

And Physician to St. Luke's Hospital.

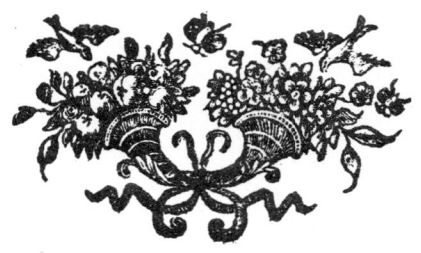

LONDON:
Printed for J. WHISTON, and B. WHITE, in Fleet-street.

M,DCC,LVIII.

[Price Two Shillings and Six-Pence.]

TO

THE MOST NOBLE

GEORGE,

Earl of CARDIGAN,

President of St. Luke's Hospital,

THIS

TREATISE on MADNESS

IS HUMBLY DEDICATED

BY

HIS LORDSHIP's

DUTIFUL AND OBLIGED SERVANT

W. BATTIE.

ADVERTISEMENT.

AMONG the many good reasons offered to the Publick, for establishing another Hospital for the reception of Lunatics, one, and that not the least considerable, was *the introducing more Gentlemen of the Faculty to the Study and Practice of one of the most important branches of Physick.*

The attention of those worthy citizens of *London*, who first planned and promoted this charitable work, was carried beyond its more immediate object. Not content with giving relief to a few indigent persons of their own age or country they interested themselves in the care of posterity; and as far as they were

were able made a more ample and effectual provision for that help, which all Lunatics of whatever nation or quality must at all times stand most in need of.

Agreeably to this their extensive benevolence, they very soon by an unanimous vote signified their inclination of admitting young Physicians well recommended to visit with me in the Hospital, and freely to observe the treatment of the patients there confined.

A command so conformable to my own sentiments I not only most readily obeyed; but, that I might answer their expectations in this as well as in every other particular to the utmost of my power, I moreover offered to the perusal of the Gentlemen who honoured me with their attendance the reasons of those prescriptions, which were submitted to their observation.

The

The end propofed in committing my thoughts to writing on this fubject has induced me to publifh. Thofe, for whofe ufe thefe papers were originally defigned, having encouraged me to hope that the fame hints may be of fervice to other Students, who have not the fame opportunity of feeing practice.

Lately Publiſhed,

By JOHN WHISTON *and* BENJ. WHITE, *in* ONE VOLUME Quarto, *Price* 12*s. Bound,*

DE PRINCIPIIS ANIMALIBUS Exercitationes viginti quatuor in Theatro Collegii Medicorum Londinenſium habitæ.

A GULIELMO BATTIE, *M. D.*

Collegii ejuſdem Socio.

——*Nunquam aliud Natura aliud Sapientia dicit.*

A TREATISE ON MADNESS.

SECT. I.

The Definition of Madness.

MADNESS, though a terrible and at present a very frequent calamity, is perhaps as little underſtood as any that ever afflicted mankind. The names alone uſually given to this diſorder and its ſeveral ſpecies, *viz. Lunacy, Spleen, Melancholy, Hurry of the Spirits,* &c. may convince any one of the truth

truth of this assertion, without having recourse to the authors who have professedly treated on this subject.

Our defect of knowledge in this matter is, I am afraid, in a great measure owing to a defect of proper communication: and the difficulties attending the care of Lunaticks have been at least perpetuated by their being entrusted to Empiricks, or at best to a few select Physicians, most of whom thought it adviseable to keep the cases as well as the patients to themselves. By which means it has unavoidably happened that in this instance experience, the parent of medical science, has profited little, and every Practitioner at his first engaging in the cure of Lunacy has had nothing but his own natural sense and sagacity to trust to; except what he may perchance have heard of Antimonial vomits, strong purges, and Hellebore, as specifically antimaniacal: Which traditional knowledge however, if indiscriminately reduced to practice, a little experience will soon make him wish he had been an entire stranger to.

There is therefore reason to hope, that an attempt to discover the causes, effects, and cure of Madness, will meet with a favourable reception; since, whatever may be the event, the intention is is right; and it is some comfort to think that nothing of this nature, even though it should fall short of what is aimed at, can in its consequences be entirely useless. For the judicious reader will at least be hereby inclined to turn his thoughts to the same subject, and may even receive instruction from the miscarriages of such an undertaking.

But the peculiar misfortune just now mentioned, *viz.* want of proper communication, though the chief, is not the only hindrance to our knowledge: for Madness hath moreover shared the fate common to many other distempers of not being precisely defined. Inasmuch as not only several symptoms, which frequently and accidentally accompany it, have been taken into the account as constant, necessary, and essential; but also the supposed cause, which perhaps never existed or certainly never acted with such effect, has been implied in the very names usually given to this distemper. No wonder therefore is it, whilst several disorders, really independent of Madness and of one another, are thus blended together in our bewildered imagination, that a treatment, rationally indicated by any of those disorders, should be injudiciously directed against Madness itself, whether attended with such symptoms or not. Much less can we blame the Physician,

sician, who being prejudiced by the supposed cause couched in the name of the distemper he has to deal with at every new or full Moon attenuates, evacuates, or alters the peccant humours by medicines peculiarly adapted to the black or splendid Bile, &c.

In order therefore to avoid this mischievous confusion of sentiment as well as language, and that we may fix a clear and determinate meaning to the Word *Madness*; we must for some time at least quit the schools of Philosophy, and content ourselves with a vulgar apprehension of things; we must reject not only every supposed cause of Madness, but also every symptom which does not necessarily belong to it, and retain no one phœnomenon but what is essential, that is without which the word *Madness* becomes nugatory and conveys no idea whatever: or, in other words, no definition of Madness can be safe, which does not, with regard at least to some particular symptoms, determine what it is not, as well as what it is.

First then, though too great and too lively a perception of objects that really exist creates an uneasiness not felt by the generality of men, and therefore discovers a præternatural state in the instruments of Sensation, and tho' such uneasiness frequently accompanies Madness, and is therefore

fore sometimes mistaken for it; nevertheless Anxiety is no more essentially annexed to Madness, so as to make part of our complex idea, than Fever, Head-ach, Gout, or Leprosy. Witness the many instances of happy Mad-men, who are perfectly easy under what is esteemed by every one but themselves the greatest misfortune human nature is liable to.

Secondly, though too little and too languid a perception of things that really exist and are obtruded with force sufficient to excite sensation in the generality of men, discovers as præternatural a state or disorder in the instruments of Sensation as uncommon Anxiety, and tho' it sometimes attends Madness, and is likewise mistaken for it, especially by the *French* who call Mad-men and Fools by the same name; nevertheless such defect of Sensation is no more essentially annexed to Madness than the former symptom of Anxiety, which that very frequent symptom of Madness sufficiently proves.

But--*qui species alias veris capiet, commotus habebitur* --- And this by all mankind as well as the Physician: no one ever doubting whether the perception of objects not really existing or not really corresponding to the senses be a certain sign of Madness. Therefore *deluded imagination*, which

which is not only an indisputable but an essential character of Madness, (that is without which, all accidental symptoms being removed from our thoughts, we have no idea whatever remaining annexed to that sound) precisely discriminates this from all other animal disorders: or that man and that man alone is properly mad, who is fully and unalterably persuaded of the Existence or of the appearance of any thing, which either does not exist or does not actually appear to him, and who behaves according to such erroneous persuasion.

Madness, or false perception, being then a præternatural state or disorder of Sensation; before we attempt to discover its causes effects and cure, it will be necessary for us to investigate the seat the causes and the effects of natural Sensation. For the consideration of the abuse or fault of any thing necessarily brings that very thing into comparison with what it was when sound and perfect; and 'tis impossible for us rationally to amend or restore what never was the object of our thoughts.

Be it therefore our first endeavour to contemplate natural Sensation : if haply this most distinguishing property of animal life may supply us with actual and positive knowledge of some matters

ters that relate to the present subject; or at least may point out to us what it is that herein surpasses our imperfect understandings. A science negative indeed, and by no means so satisfactory to the pride and speculative curiosity of man as the former, but very often as useful and as conducive to the attaining practical truth.

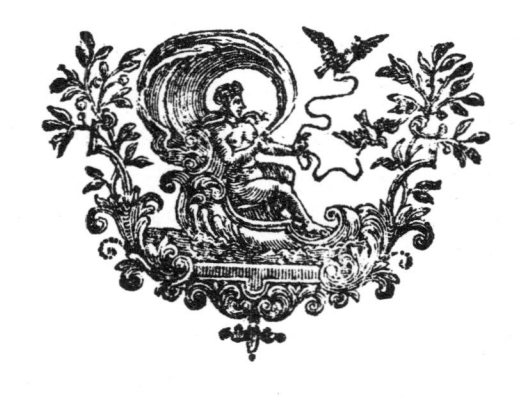

SECT.

SECT. II.

The Seat of natural Sensation.

Whoever is conscious that he hears, sees, or feels, and beholds all animals he is conversant with acting just in the same manner as he does when he hears, sees, or feels, must acknowledge that his own and every other animal body is as really endued with Sensation as that it exists.

Whoever attentively contemplates in what manner he and every other animal is affected by external impulse, must acknowledge that some parts of the same body, however animated, are quite insensible, some endued with a less degree of Sensation than others.

Whoever is moreover sufficiently versed in Anatomical researches, and has learnt to separate those parts of an animal body, which, however contiguous or closely connected, are nevertheless really distinct from each other, very readily discovers several soft fibres, each of which is actually divisible into many smaller of the same kind, as far as his eye can trace; and he by analogy justly concludes that each of those smaller fibres

is

is as capable of being still farther and farther divided beyond the reach of vision, and even of human imagination.

These soft fibres are all connected with the contents of the cranium, and in different parts of the body they are collected into fasciculi; every one of which is enveloped by a continuation of those very membranes which within the cranium contain the substance of the brain and its medullary appendages.

Every such fasciculus as well as the several fibres it is resolveable into is called *a Nerve:* a name borrowed indeed from the ancients, but used by them in a very different signification. For by νεῦρον and *nervus* neither the *Greeks* nor *Latins* meant any thing soft and medullary, but on the contrary the hard and elastic substance of a tendon or ligament; as the word ἀπονεύρωσις, still retained by the moderns to signify the fascia or membrane expanded over and connecting the muscular fibres, sufficiently shews.

Every nerve, which is within the reach of our observation, is extended between the *medulla oblongata* or its appendage the *medulla spinalis* and the place of such nerve's destination. But every such nerve is thus extended in a manner

ner very different from the difpofition of the blood-veffels, and indeed of all other portions of the fame body which are called fimilar. For in its paffage it neither is fplit into ramifications, nor is it at all connected with any contiguous parts of the body, except with fome fubftances equally nervous called ganglions chiefly obfervable in the mefentery.

If a nerve in a living body be diftracted by external force, there immediately arifes an exquifite fenfation called pain. Which fenfation is always in a direct proportion to the quantity of fuch diftracting force; and which never ceafes either untill the diftracting force is removed or is become unactive, or untill the material particles which conftitute the faid nerve are by this diftraction irrecoverably difunited.

If to a nerve in a living body be applied any acrimonious objects, that is fuch portions of matter whofe furfaces are full of angles, and which when affifted with proper impulfe are therefore capable of diftracting the particles that conftitute the nervous fubftance, there immediately arifes the fame painful fenfation: which is always in a direct proportion to the quantity and acutenefs of fuch acrimonious angles, and to the impulfe with which they are impacted, and which continues

tinues as long as in the former cafe of vifible diftraction occafioned by external force.

Thofe parts of an animal body, in which the greateft quantity of nervous fibres is manifeftly contained, and in which fuch nervous fibres lie the moft expofed and undefended by any other matter that conftitutes the fame body, are the fooneft and the moft affected whenever any external objects are applied with force fufficient to excite fenfation.

Thofe membranes, which not only within the cranium furround the brain, but which alfo ferve as fheaths to the feveral appendages of the brain, collecting them into nervous fafciculi all over the body as far as the eye can trace, are indeed every where contiguous to and feem intimately connected with the medullary fubftance they contain: neverthelefs upon the application of any external objects they all difcover no extraordinary figns of fenfibility, any more than feveral other membranes in the fame body, which are equally vafcular and elaftic. Witnefs the many well attefted cafes of erofions and other accidents of the dura mater unattended with any degree of pain.

All which constant and uncontroverted observations prove, 1. That the nervous or medullary substance derived from or rather communicating with the brain is the seat or instrument of natural Sensation: 2. That no other matter whatever, whether animated or not, is such seat or instrument.

SECT. III.

The supposed Causes of natural Sensation.

THAT the medullary or nervous substance continued from or rather connected with the brain is the seat of Sensation, is a point now so universally agreed upon, that perhaps it might have been sufficient barely to have asserted it without any formal proof. Happy should we be, if the causes of Sensation were as clearly and incontestably settled.

But I am afraid before any right or satisfactory notion can be formed concerning this matter, we must get rid of some opinions, which however absurd have of late passed upon many for real knowledge.

The reason of this difference, which at present subsists between the discovery of the seat, and the discovery of the causes of Sensation, is not in the things themselves that have been enquired after, but in the manner of enquiry. Because in fixing the seat of Sensation we have been content with facts that are apparent to all men, and which if any one should controvert, he must disclaim the evidence of his own senses:
But

But in assigning the causes of Sensation several things have been assumed as matters of fact, which have never been discovered, and which may at least with equal probability be denied as admitted.

For here the Hypothetical Genius, forgetful that he hath Nature's works for his contemplation, and despising that poor pittance of knowledge which the real appearance of things supplies every one with as well as himself, hath dared without any warrant to coin new ideas; hath made free with air, water, æther, nay even electrical fire; and imagining that to be probable which is barely possible, and then heightening this assumed probability up to matter of fact, he takes one large stride more and roundly asserts that *the brain is a gland; that its cortical portion is a convolution of secretory vessels designed to separate from the blood one or other of those elementary substances, which he hath by ways unknown introduced into the carotid arteries for this his present purpose; that the medullary portion of the brain and nerves is nothing else but a collection of excretory ducts serving to convey this elementary matter to all the sensible parts of the body: which matter either by undulation or retrograde motion imparts to the Sensorium commune all those impulses it receives from such external objects as affect*

affect the extremities of the nervous filaments. This excrement therefore of the brain tho' invisible is the necessary cause of sight, tho' impalpable the sufficient cause of feeling, and tho' an animal Spirit the material cause of animal Sensation.

Now, as the secretion of such a nervous fluid and consequently its very existence depends entirely upon the analogy that is supposed to lie between the brain and every glandular substance, in case the brain is very unlike a gland in any material circumstance, this whole machinery is immediately destroyed.

Admitting therefore, what has never yet been proved, that the cortical portion of the brain resembles the secretory organ of a gland, yet the medullary or nervous substance is different from all excretory ducts whatever: inasmuch as no excretory duct is ever found but what is immediately detached from the gland whence it issues; whereas on the contrary the supposed glandular or secretory substance of the brain is continued to every part supplied with nerves, and these nerves the supposed excretory ducts, after that they have left the cranium and their glandular origin the brain, wherever they are capable of being examined, remain as closely connected

not

not only with the cortical or secretory portion of the brain, but even with the productions of the dura and pia mater, as the medullary substance itself whilst contained within the cranium.

This observation alone would be sufficient to destroy the very foundation of a nervous fluid, if any Hypothesis whatever could deserve a serious consideration. But it may be feared that a solemn confutation of chimæras will appear equally ridiculous as an attempt to establish them; and he may perhaps incur the suspicion of insanity which these theorists have deserved, who shall fight in earnest with shadows, and mispend his time in offering reasons, why the solid constituent parts of the medullary substance contained in every nerve bid fairer for supplying us with the material cause of Sensation, than a fluid never yet discovered, and which its very authors confess was once foreign to the body, and even extracted from dead and putrescent matter spirited up, we know not how, into animality.

Let us therefore quit this enchanted ground to those, if such there be, who are still inclined to dispute upon it; and in order to clear our way a little more to the real causes of Sensation, let us divert our attention to a very common phrase, *viz. weakness of nerves*, which tho' not professedly

feſſedly ſyſtematical, like the former ſcheme of *animal ſpirits*, is neverthelefs extremely deluſive; inaſmuch as it ſeems indirectly to offer another ſolution of the phœnomenon in queſtion, and to aſcertain the cauſe of Senſation.

For ſince the word *weakneſs*, when joined with material ſubſtances, can convey no idea but a lax cohæſion of ſuch particles as conſtitute thoſe ſubſtances; therefore the phraſe *weakneſs of nerves*, which denotes a morbid exceſs of Senſation, ſeems to imply that Senſation itſelf is owing to the looſe cohæſion of thoſe material particles which conſtitute the nervous ſubſtance, inaſmuch as the quantity of every effect muſt be proportionable to its cauſe.

By this inaccurate manner of talking, the moſt diſtinguiſhing property of animal nature is in danger of being blended with inanimate matter. For, if the caſe really were what theſe words ſeem to import, all bodies whoſe particles do not cohære with too great a degree of proximity would be nervous, that is endued with Senſation. But, ſince no portion of matter, however looſely compacted, is nervous except it is part of an animal body, therefore the medullary ſubſtance of a nerve is endued with Senſation not becauſe its conſtituent particles are looſely united:

and every nervous filament, tho' it confifts of parts extended and not too clofely cohæring, is confeffedly as diftinct from every other material fubftance confifting of parts extended and equally cohæring, as a man from a carcas, or an horfe from an equeftrian ftatue.

SECT. IV.

The real Causes of natural Sensation.

SENSATION, however perplexed it may seem to those who too curiously enquire into its nature, is to the modest observer as clear in idea and as fully to be accounted for, at least to all useful intents and purposes, as any phœnomenon whatever.

For is not what we feel a plain matter of fact, of which we are not only certain and conscious ourselves, but which we are likewise capable of communicating to others by words or signs? And are we not perfectly well acquainted with many things, which when impelled with force sufficient will make us feel; and which it is frequently in our power to apply, remove, or avoid, as best suits our interest?

It is the heedless or rather the wilful neglect of precisely separating these many evident and external causes of Sensation as well from their unknown and internal operations as from their intermediate and equally unknown effects, that has created such difficulties in contemplating this phœnomenon.

For the mutual cohæsion of material particles, as essential to our idea of an animal body as sense itself, but not better accounted for, hath however been looked upon as a thing much less mysterious.

Which seeming diversity can be owing to nothing else, but because the generality of mankind have contented themselves with the useful and the attainable knowledge of such external objects, as will harden or soften those bodies they are applied to, without enquiring too nicely why the constituent particles of those bodies are more or less united upon such application, or indeed why they are united at all: whereas the philosopher in his contemplation of sensible matter is not content with knowing certainly like other men what objects externally applied to a nerve will create, increase, or deaden sensation, but moreover conjectures why; and attempts by any means whatever to assign the manner in which these external objects act upon, and the changes they produce in the nervous substance previous to sensation their last effect; which effect, for reasons best known to himself, seems to demand a more explicit solution than the cohæsion of material particles.

In

In endeavouring therefore to assign the causes of Sensation, be it one of our chiefest cares to distinguish them from one another as effectually in our mind, as they are really different in their nature, and to separate what we actually and usefully know from what we are, and perhaps shall always be without any great damage, entirely ignorant of.

For which purpose, it may not be amiss to premise a few considerations on causes in general; which will illustrate the subject of our present enquiry and at the same time be confirmed thereby.

First then, by observing that any one phœnomenon frequently follows another, we conclude that the second is owing to the first; and hence we get the ideas of *cause* and *effect*.

Secondly, by observing that any one phœnomenon never fails to follow another, we conclude that the first is not only a cause but also a sufficient cause of the second.

Thirdly, by observing that the second phœnomenon never occurs but in consequence of the first, we further conclude that the first is not only

only a cause but a necessary cause of the second, which is therefore called the *causa sine qua non*.

Fourthly, by observing that the second phœnomenon follows the first without either the evident or the demonstrated intervention of any other phœnomenon as necessary or at least accessary to its existence, we conclude that the first phœnomenon is moreover the immediate cause of the second.

Fifthly, by observing either that the first phœnomenon is not always succeeded by the second, or that the second is not always preceded by the first, we conclude that the first phœnomenon is either not a sufficient or not a necessary, but merely an accidental cause of the second.

Sixthly, by observing or by admitting as undeniable that any one or more phœnomena intervene between the first and the last in question, we plainly discover that the first is remote, and that the several other intervening phœnomena in their order approach nearer and nearer to the immediate cause.

Seventhly, a very little reflection upon causes and effects as thus stated will make us conclude that the remote and accidental causes of any effect

effect may be many, but that the sufficient and necessary as well as the immediate cause can be but one. Since either of two causes supposed sufficient will render the other unnecessary; and either cause supposed necessary will render the other insufficient. Which unavoidable conclusion, by the way, might be extended beyond secondary agents or instruments, improperly called causes, and would give an additional proof, if any was wanting, to the unity of the first, the necessary, the sufficient, and indeed strictly speaking the sole cause of all things.

Thus, to instance in our present subject; sight, hearing, taste, smell, &c. which frequently succeed the application of external objects, are looked upon by us as the effects of such external objects; and we in common discourse refer our ideas back to those objects as to their causes, as when we say *we see the sun, we hear the drum,* &c.

But, forasmuch as the external objects of sense, however forcible their application may be, do not always and in all animal bodies create sight, &c. And moreover, as the very same perceptions do sometimes, at least in disordered subjects, arise without any external object that really affects them; it is impossible but every such external object must be meerly accidental, and by no means

means the sufficient or the necessary cause of such its nervous effect: Which sufficient and necessary cause is therefore internal, that is it inhæres in the very frame and constitution of the nervous substance itself; whereby alone such substance is rendered capable of being affected by any external object so as to create Sensation; and without which internal cause no thing whatever would actually become an object of our senses.

For the same reason all such external causes are not only accidental but likewise remote. Since the necessary and sufficient cause at least must intervene; and besides, before an external object can create any sensation whatever, it must produce several intermediate effects, *viz.* motion, impulse, and pressure: all which precede not only sight, *&c.* thereby excited, but also precede that particular internal affection of the nerve itself, whatever it is, which is the immediate, the necessary, and the sufficient cause of such perception.

The accidental and remote causes of Sensation, as also their intermediate effects, provided such effects are external to the nervous substance, very readily discover themselves, and are clearly comprehended. For indeed they are all bodies

bodies that lye within our obfervation (many of which are within our reach) and the motion and impulfe of thofe bodies, or of particles emitted therefrom, upon the organs of fenfe: which every one not only has a clear idea of, but is moreover certain of their exiftence, motion, and impulfe.

Now, as no body whatever can be capable of creating Senfation in confequence of its motion and impulfe, without preffing upon the nerve affected by fuch impulfe; therefore preffure of the medullary fubftance contained in the nervous filaments approaches nearer in order to the immediate caufe of Senfation, than the motion and impulfe of any external object.

Preffure of the medullary fubftance contained in the nervous filaments cannot indeed be imagined without fome alteration in the former arrangement of thofe material particles which conftitute that fubftance. But we have no idea whatever, either vifible or intellectual, how and in what manner thofe particles are by fuch preffure differently juxtapofited, previoufly to Senfation thereby excited.

Whence it undeniably follows that preffure upon the medullary fubftance contained in the nervous

nervous filaments is the laſt in order of all thoſe cauſes of Senſation, which we have any idea of. Thus far and no farther our knowledge in theſe matters reaches, limited by the outſide of the ſeat of Senſation; what paſſes within being meer conjecture. For if a new poſition of medullary particles, which is an immediate and unavoidable effect of external preſſure, does not diſcover itſelf any more than their conſtitutional arrangement; what account can we with any the leaſt degree of modeſty pretend to give of all the alterations in the nervous ſubſtance ſtill ſubſequent to ſuch preſſure and to change of place thereby occaſioned; a regular ſeries of which may, for any thing we know to the contrary, precede the immediate cauſe of ſenſation.

SECT.

SECT. V.

The salutary Effects of natural Sensation.

SENSATION is always accompanied with some degree of pleasure or uneasiness; no animal being indifferent to what he sees, hears, or feels. These additional and in some degree inseparable affections demonstrate the direct tendency of Sensation to the preservation of life; inasmuch as every one spontaneously flies from those objects which hurt and are at enmity with him, and covets such as create satisfaction and are suitable to his interest.

But, tho' no one at first sight would doubt whether the perception of pleasure is agreeable to his nature, and conducive to its preservation; it may with great reason be doubted by those who reflect a little whether such perception, however convenient it may seem to animal life, is alone instrumental in its preservation, and without the intervention of the contrary affection ever conduces to health.

For uneasiness is so interwoven in the very frame of mortals, that even the greatest present satis-

satisfaction implies the removing or stifling the greatest uneasiness which before disquieted. And a sense of future pleasure, as it excites desire, in that very desire implies a present uneasiness adequate to the supposed enjoyment of the pleasure in expectation. By which present uneasiness, according to Mr. *Locke*'s just observation, the will is determined.

However paradoxical therefore it may seem, nothing is more true than that Anxiety, a real evil, is nevertheless productive of real good; and, tho' seemingly disagreeable to Nature, is absolutely necessary to our preservation, in such a manner, that without its severe but useful admonitions the several species of animals would speedily be destroyed.

For first, are not hunger and thirst very salutary Anxieties? By which the nerves of the mouth œsophagus and stomach excite all animals from the first moment of their birth to seize on such objects, as are capable of relieving those natural and healthy but agonizing sensations.

Now the real good produced by the gratification of these appetites is by no means to be placed in their present gratification alone. Whatever he may imagine, who being ignorant of the animal

animal œconomy looks no farther than the actual pleafure which accompanies the ftifling fuch fenfations. For the end herein propofed by the Author of Nature is undoubtedly the refection of that very body which hungers and thirfts; whofe conftituent particles by the inevitable effects of vital action are in a continual flux and decay; whereas the efficient or coercive caufes of eating and drinking are thofe fenfations alone, which torment every animal to a very good purpofe. Who perhaps would not otherwife give himfelf the trouble of opening his mouth, much lefs by hard labour earn food wherewith to fill it; even tho' he fhould be affured that the lofs of meat and drink to-day, tho' not at all inconvenient to him at prefent, will be fenfibly felt to-morrow by his diftempered body, and that his idlenefs and fafting will be foon attended by fatal confequences.

Secondly, the introducing frefh air into the lungs being as neceffary for the immediate continuance of life, as it is for other purpofes of the animal œconomy which are more remote, and at prefent unknown; therefore every animal provided with organs of refpiration, whether awake or fleeping, draws into his breaft and expels a quantity of external air fufficient to diftend them from the firft moment of his birth till

till the laſt period of life. Which alternate action, if he either careleſsly or obſtinately omits it, he is very ſoon compelled to perform by that inexpreſſible Anxiety which attends a long detention of air once admitted as well as the refuſing admiſſion to any air at all.

Thirdly, foraſmuch as voluntary exerciſe of the body is no leſs requiſite to the due circulation and ſecretions of the animal fluids, and the ſalutary conſequences thereon depending, than the propulſive action of the heart and the reſilition of the arterial tubes; which the ill effects of a ſedentary life ſufficiently prove; therefore the uneaſy ſenſation that is always occaſioned by ſatiety and the weariſome condition of idleneſs determine all animals, to whom activity is thus neceſſary, frequently to alter their place of reſidence, and to remove from thoſe objects they have long been converſant with, however pleaſing and eagerly ſought for they might once have been.

Fourthly, all the afore-mentioned inſtances of uneaſy ſenſation, however nearly allied to and often ending in ſickneſs, are nevertheleſs the natural effects of perfect health. But beſides theſe there occur ſeveral other anxieties, which are the unavoidable effects of real ſickneſs and

and moreover frequently determine the will of the patient to such things as are capable either of relieving the present disorder or of preventing its mischievous consequences. Thus, to instance in one particular, feaverish heat threatens putrid obstructions, and at the same time occasions intense thirst and an almost insatiable craving for acidulated water. Which desire, if not contradicted by the officious and ill-tim'd care of the by-standers, procures a remedy that is both diluting and antiseptic.

Lastly, tho' the nervous energy be neither absolutely necessary nor alone sufficient to excite muscular action, yet such is the connection between the nervous and muscular fibres, however really distinct from each other, that animal sensation often instantaneously precedes animal action, so as to have confounded these two qualities, or at least to have made the one appear the immediate and only cause of the other. And, what chiefly deserves our notice whilst we are considering the salutary effects of Sensation, Convulsion itself, a distempered excess of animal motion, which is a frequent effect of uneasy Sensation, sometimes becomes its sudden and efficacious remedy, by removing the material cause of such uneasy Sensation, and that without any

any determination or interposition of the will whatever.

All which nervous appetites as well as muscular motions, that either preserve or restore health, and are seemingly excited by somewhat rationally forecasting their salutary ends, have given rise, I suppose, to some modern metaphorical expressions, *viz. Nature,* and the *Anima* invented by *Willis* and deifyed by *Stahl.* Which figurative words, tho' not quite philosophical, are innocent and even useful, in case they are applied only to avoid periphrases in relating medical matters of fact. But young Practitioners, who are often told that they are to imitate and assist Nature, must take great care not to be misguided by the literal sense of words, or fancy any thing like personal consciousness and intellectual agency in the animal œconomy. For in such case of misapprehension these and the like expressions become as absurd as all the exploded *Faculties of the Ancients,* and, what is much worse, may be as mischievous as an instrument of death in the hands of a Madman.

SECT.

SECT. VI.

The Causes and Effects of Anxiety and Insensibility, two species of Sensation disordered tho' not delusive.

HAVING contemplated the feat causes and effects of natural and true Sensation; before we proceed to consider delusive Sensation, the only subject of this enquiry, it may be not improper to take some notice of those two other disorders of the same quality, which were excluded from our definition of Madness, *viz.* præternatural *Anxiety* or Sensation too greatly excited by real objects, and its contrary *Insensibility* or Sensation not sufficiently excited by real objects, tho' acting with their usual force and tho' capable of engaging the attention of all other healthy animals of the same species.

For, although Madness in its proper sense be clearly distinct from the too lively or the too languid perception of things really existing, it however very often is preceded by or accompanied with the first and as often terminates in the second of these two disorders. Besides the being too much affected by external impulse, tho' it does

does by no means imply Senſation materially deluſive, inaſmuch as the ideas excited by ſuch impulſe are referred to true and correſponding objects; yet the quantity of concomitant affection not being proportionate and therefore not in all reſpects correſponding to the natural quantity of its real cauſe hath apparently ſome deviation from abſolute truth, and from the natural and uſual circumſtances of this animal function. And Senſation not proportionate to real impulſe, tho' it is not ſtrictly ſpeaking deluſive, hath however as great a deviation from abſolute truth as exceſſive Senſation itſelf.

Now Senſation, which in its moſt natural and perfect ſtate is ſooner or later attended with ſome degree of uneaſineſs, may with very little addition be heightened into Anxiety either by the too great or too long continued force of external objects, or by the illconditioned ſtate of the nerve itſelf, whereby it is rendered liable to be too much affected with the uſual action of ſuch external objects.

This illconditioned ſtate of the nerve may be inhærent in the internal proper and unknown conſtitution of the medullary ſubſtance, or it may be external to that ſubſtance, and ariſe from the loſs or defect of thoſe membranes which envelope

velope and sheathe the seat of Sensation, and are designed to protect it from such rude attacks and impressions as might otherwise endanger the dissolution of so soft a matter.

For, whenever those integuments are quite removed from a nerve which is endued with no more than a common share of sensibility, Anxiety must ensue the application of any external objects that are capable of exciting natural Sensation. And in fact we find that the laying bare any sensible part and exposing it to the common air, which usually refreshes the body whilst cloathed with skin, immediately distracts us with intolerable torment.

For the same reason Anxiety, which follows an entire removal of the nervous sheaths, will in some degree arise whenever those sheaths are not strong and sufficiently compacted so as to answer the purpose of defence. That is the sensation of the nervous or medullary fibres, tho' they continue the same, will be in a reverse proportion to the cohæsion of those minute particles which constitute the solid and elastic fibres. And in fact we find that Anxiety is almost always the consequence of morbid laxity, except where the intervention of fat, lymph, or viscid congestions owing

owing to such laxity substitute an occasional defence.

No wonder is it then that the straining or loosening the solid parts of human bodies should frequently render those bodies liable to be violently affected by such objects as are scarce felt or attended to by other men, who enjoy a natural or artificial strength and compactness of fibres.

And from hence we are enabled to annex a true and intelligible meaning to that expression before taken notice of, *viz. weakness of nerves*. Which word *weakness* would not have been so improper, if it had been joined in idea not to that substance which is strictly nervous, but to its integuments and contiguous membranes; and if laxity, an accidental and remote cause of excessive and therefore uneasy Sensation, had not been thereby made liable to be mistaken for its immediate necessary and sufficient cause.

Whatever may be the cause of Anxiety, it chiefly discovers itself by that agonising impatience observable in some men of black *November* days, of easterly winds, of heat, cold, damps, &c. Which real misery of theirs is sometimes derided by duller mortals as a whimsical affectation.
And

And of the same nature are the perpetual tempests of love, hatred, and other turbulent passions provoked by nothing or at most by very trifles. In which state of habitual diseases many drag on their wretched lives; whilst others, unequal to evils of which they see no remedy but death, rashly resolve to end them at any rate. Which very frequent cases of suicide, though generally ascribed to Lunacy by the verdict of a good-natured Jury, except where the deceased hath not left assets, are no more entitled to the benefit of passing for pardonable acts of madness, than he who deliberately has killed the man he hated deserves to be acquitted as not knowing what he did.

Among the morbid effects of Anxiety or the præternatural excess of Sensation one, which frequently attends upon it and more particularly demands our attention, is Spasm or the præternatural excess of muscular action. Which state of morbid motion, tho' sometimes salutary as has been before observed, is oftner occasioned by this nervous disorder to no good purpose whatever; and, when very violent or of long continuance, is necessarily productive of numberless evils and of acute and chronical distempers, which if not relieved in time almost always end in death.

Another

Another effect of Anxiety or of the præternatural excess of Sensation is the nervous disorder directly contrary to it, *viz.* Insensibility, that is a præternatural defect or total loss of Sensation.

Whether this entire change from one extream to the other is owing to the material instruments of Sensation having been strained by Anxiety or rather by some of its causes, cannot perhaps be determined with any degree of certainty. But thus much is clear in reason that any distraction, which is sufficient to disunite or break in pieces the medullary substance, must be sufficient to make it unfit for its function; and it is as undeniable in fact that Anxiety is frequently either attended with such spasmodic disorders or occasioned by such external injuries as must necessarily distract the nerves thereby affected.

Not that Insensibility is owing to no other cause except Anxiety. For it is at least as often occasioned by the internal and unknown constitution of the nervous or medullary substance itself, which was either formed imperfect at first or hath since degenerated.

And

And, besides the internal and unknown defect in the seat of Sensation, Insensibility may as often be ascribed to another cause external to the nerve and sufficiently understood. For, since the nervous integuments or neighbouring membranes do sheathe the medullary substance, and thereby prevent the morbid excess of its energy; whenever the fibres that compose those integuments or membranes are præternaturally compacted and of too close a texture, instead of moderating they undoubtedly must deaden or destroy Sensation. And for the same reason those nerves that are pillowed with fat, soaked in lymph, or stifled by obstructed vessels, cannot and in fact do not receive a proper that is a sensible impulse from external objects, altho' such objects are rightly and forcibly applied, and although the nervous substance itself is perfectly sound, and in its internal constitution fitted for the efficacious reception of such external impulse.

But, whatever may be the cause of Insensibility, its ill effects are many and as obvious as they are unavoidable, and need not be here enumerated. For they are all those disorders in the animal œconomy, which Sensation in its natural vigour was designed to prevent. The
defect

defect therefore or loss of this salutary and vital quality must either hurry on or suffer the sickly body to approach nearer and nearer to the last period of animal life.

SECT.

SECT. VII.

The Causes of Madness.

Whoever is satisfied with our account of the seat and causes of natural and true Sensation, will acknowledge that the one immediate necessary and sufficient cause of the præternatural and false perception of objects, which either do not exist, or which do not in this instance excite such sensation, must be some disorder of that substance which is medullary and strictly nervous. And moreover, as he cannot discover the natural and internal constitution of this medullary substance, which renders it fit for the proper perception of real and external impulse or rather of the ideas thereby excited; he must for the same reason own that he is unable to discover wherein consists that præternatural and internal state of the same nervous matter, which disposes it to be without any such impulse affected by those very ideas, that would have been presented to the imagination, if the same nervous matter had been acted upon by something external. Or, to speak more technically, forasmuch as the one immediate necessary and sufficient cause of the perception of real objects is unknown, we must likewise remain entirely ignorant of the one immediate necessary and sufficient cause of the perception of Chimæras, which exist no where except in the brain of a Madman.

But, altho' the immediate and internal cause of delusive as well as of true Sensation is absolutely hid, many remoter and external causes thereof frequently discover themselves to the by-stander, notwithstanding that the idea thus excited is not by the patient himself referred to any one of those true causes, but to something else, which may or may not exist, and which certainly does not in this particular case act upon the affected organ.

Thus, to instance in a very common accident, the eye that is violently struck immediately sees flames flash before it; which idea of fire presented to the imagination plainly shews that those material particles which constitute the medullary substance of the optic nerve are affected by such blow exactly in the same manner, as they are when real fire acts upon the eye of a man awake and in his senses with force sufficient to provoke his attention. Thus variety of sounds disturb the ear that is shocked by the pulsation of vessels, by the inflammation or other

obstruction

obstruction of those membranes which line the *meatus auditorius*, by the intrusion of water, and in short by any material force external to the medullary portion of the seventh pair of nerves; which force hath no connection with any sonorous body, that by its elastic vibration communicates an undulatory motion to the intermediate air.

Now suppose that any one perfectly awake without the accident of such a blow sees fire, or without the pulsation of vessels, inflammation, or any obstruction in the *meatus auditorius, &c.* hears sounds; or suppose that the idea of flame really excited by a blow is by him referred to an house on fire, or the idea of sound excited by the pulsation of vessels, *&c.* is referred to a musical instrument, which is not near enough to be heard, or is not really played upon; the man who is so mistaken, and who cannot be set right either upon his own recollection or the information of those about him, is in the apprehension of all sober persons a Lunatic.

From whence we may collect that Madness with respect to its cause is distinguishable into two species. The first is solely owing to an internal disorder of the nervous substance: the second is likewise owing to the same nervous substance being indeed in like manner difordered, but difordered *ab extra*; and therefore is chiefly to be attributed to fome remote and accidental caufe. The firft fpecies, until a better name can be found, may be called *Original*, the fecond may be called *Confequential Madnefs*.

The internal diforder of the medullary fubftance, or the caufe of Original Madnefs, for the fame reafon as the immediate neceffary and fufficient caufe of true Senfation, can be but one: but the external and accidental caufes of Confequential Madnefs, as well as of true Senfation, may be many.

Now no external caufe whatever can be fuppofed capable of exciting delufive any more than true perception, except fuch caufe acts materially upon the nerve thereby difordered, and that with force fufficient to alter the former arrangement of its medullary particles. Which force neceffarily implies impulfe and preffure in delufive Senfation, in the fame manner and order as it does in the perception of objects really correfponding thereto.

Preffure therefore amongft all the external and difcoverable caufes of falfe as well as of true perception is in our apprehenfion the neareft to fuch its apparent effect. As to the intermediate alterations

terations of the medullary substance, that may really precede delusive Sensation, they are all as much unknown as are the nervous effects which intervene between the pressure made by any external object and the true and adequate idea of that very object.

But, altho' Consequential Madness cannot be supposed without some sort and degree of pressure upon the nerves, nevertheless every sort and degree of pressure does not always and unavoidably produce Consequential Madness. For the nerves may suffer external impulse, and yet the pressure thereby occasioned either may not have force sufficient to excite any idea at all; or it may act with too great a force and in so shocking a manner as to dissolve or greatly disunite the medullary matter; in which case Sensation, which can never exist but whilst that matter does properly cohere, instead of being perverted will be abolished, or at least suspended untill the constituent particles are reunited.

What this particular sort and degree of pressure is, which is capable of creating delusive Sensation, we are not able to ascertain; because the different circumstances of the unknown subject acted upon will make the nervous effects variable and oftentimes contrary, notwithstanding the action

tion of the known cauſe conſidered *per ſe* is in all reſpects the ſame.

But, altho' we cannot exactly deſcribe the particular ſtrength of that external impulſe which excites, any more than we can diſcover why it excites deluſive ideas; thus much we may reaſonably conclude in general that all material objects, which by their action or reſiſtance occaſion a ſufficient but not too great a preſſure upon the medullary ſubſtance contained in the nerves, may be the remoter cauſes of Conſequential Madneſs.

Which concluſion is not only agreeable to reaſon, but is moreover confirmed by matter of fact and almoſt every day's experience. Witneſs the internal exoſtoſes of the cranium, the indurations of the ſinus's and proceſſes of the Dura Mater, which have frequently been found in thoſe who died mad; witneſs the intropreſſion of the ſkull or concuſſion of the head, which if not apoplectic is almoſt always attended with a delirium. And indeed every one, who contemplates ſeveral caſes of Conſequential Madneſs and thoſe accidents which precede the ſame, will find that preſſure of the medullary ſubſtance ſomewhere or other collected intervenes between ſuch accidents and theſe their delirious effects.

One

One case of Consequential Madness that proves the intervention of such pressure is an effect of Insolation or what the *French* call *coup du Soleil*. An instance of which I lately met with in a Sailor, who became raving mad in a moment while the Sun beams darted perpendicularly upon his head. Which maniacal effect of heat could be attributed to no assignable cause, except either to the violent impression of the Sun's rays upon the medullary substance of the brain, which the cranium in this case was not able to defend, or to the intermediate rarefaction of blood contained in the vessels of the Dura or Pia Mater, which vessels being suddenly distended compressed the same medullary substance. Of the same nature and owing to the same rarefaction of fluids in the brain are those delirious fevers called Calentures; one of which was, I suppose, mistaken for the plague by the *Author of the *Physicians last Legacy*, and treated with bleeding *usque ad animi deliquium*, which indeed is its only cure.

Another case of Consequential Madness is a sudden inflammation arising in those membranes which surround and therefore when thus distended compress the contents of the cranium and its nervous appendages. This state of inflammation whilst

* Dr. *Dover*.

whilft the patient lives difcovers itfelf by the fudden rednefs of the eyes external coat, which is a part or rather a production of the Dura Mater: and that membrane after death is frequently upon diffection found turgid and difcoloured with a red bloody fuffufion, juft in the fame manner as if it had been artificially injected.

Another cafe of Confequential Madnefs is a gradual congeftion of ferum or other fluid matter upon the fame membranes which envelop the medullary fubftance; whereby thofe membranes, tho' not with equal danger as when they are fuddenly inflamed, yet with the fame delirious effects comprefs their nervous contents. This ferous congeftion is difcoverable by the opaque and cloudy appearance of the cornea, for the fame reafon as an inflammatory tumor in the Dura Mater is betrayed by the external coat of the eye being tinged with blood.

Preffure of the medullary fubftance, the neareft in our apprehenfion to Madnefs of all its known and remoter caufes, moft frequently and moft effectually produces this its nervous effect, whilft it acts upon the contents of the cranium, as is evident from the cafes above-mentioned. But, altho' the brain is undoubtedly the principal feat of delufive fenfation, neverthelefs it is not

not the only one: forasmuch as the same sanguinary or serous obstructions are capable in any other nervous part of the body of exciting false ideas as well as in the brain, at least to some degree and in proportion to the quantity of medullary matter there collected so as to be sufficiently compressed by such obstructions. Thus the stomach, intestines, and uterus, are frequently the real seats of Madness, occasioned by the contents of these viscera being stopt in such a manner as to compress the many nervous filaments, which here communicate with one another by the mesenteric ganglia, and which enrich the contents of the abdomen with a more exquisite sensation. Thus the glutton who goes to-bed upon a full stomach is hagridden in his sleep. Thus

Men prove with child as powerful fancy works:

And patients truly hypochondriacal or hysterical refer that load of uneasiness they feel in their bellies to some imaginary object, which if it really existed and acted upon their senses would excite the very same idea.

H   SECT.

SECT. VIII.

The Causes of Madness.

FOrasmuch as præternatural pressure upon the nerves is in human apprehension the nearest to delusive sensation thereby excited; whatever injury creates such pressure must be a remoter cause of Consequential Madness.

Under this head therefore of remoter causes are to be ranked the internal exostoses of the cranium, the induration of the Dura Mater, the fracture and intropression of the skull and concussion of the head, as also, if it were of any service in the cure of madness to enumerate them, the many and various accidents these delirious injuries may be owing to.

To the same number of remoter causes we must add morbid distensions of the vessels contiguous to the medullary substance. And, as several cases mentioned in the foregoing section are clearly resolvable into such distensions, whose removal or diminution will frequently be sufficient to answer our intention and is almost always necessary and serviceable in the cure of this distemper;

per; it may be of use to spend a little time in examining into the nature and origin of those vascular distensions which end in Consequential Madness.

Whoever has attended to the accidents that animal bodies are liable to must have observed that several membranes, which in their natural state appear smooth and even, are sometimes suddenly at other times gradually elevated beyond the surface or plane they before helped to compose. To the first of these two cases writers on Surgery have given the name of *Tumors by Fluxion*, to the second that of *Tumors by Congestion*; thereby ascribing the quick or slow appearance of these swellings to the different motion of the fluids themselves, which materially formed them, and which according to the medical philosophy then in fashion contained all the resources of life health and sickness.

Now, altho' the discovery of the blood's circulation hath demonstrated that the fluids are passive in every circumstance of animal life whether sound or distempered, it will however be very useful in prosecuting the present enquiry to take into our account the cases themselves as distinguished from one another by their different manner of appearance which cannot be controverted,

verted, and then endeavour to assign other reasons for such their appearance, which not only really exist, but which also are sufficient to produce either species of tumor.

Tumors then by Fluxion ending in Madness are either vessels distended by the rarefaction of their proper and natural contents, as in the case of Insolation; or, which is the most frequent accident, they are the same vessels obstructed by the sudden intrusion of improper fluids into smaller canals which were never designed to give either a passage or admittance to such contents, as in the case of Inflammation. Now this change of place and forcible propulsion of fluids from their natural ducts into improper receptacles must apparently be owing to some power external to the fluids so propelled, which power either was not excited or did not effectually act the moment before such delirious obstructions took place. But the spasmodic constriction of those muscular fibres which surround the extremities of arteries and veins, and are at rest till ruffled by some accident, is a power occasionally excited, and when acting with sufficient force is capable of driving the blood out of its natural channels into vessels not originally fitted for its reception. And it is moreover a repeated observation that Madness frequently succeeds or accompanies Fever, Epilepsy,

Epilepsy, Child-birth, and the like muscular disorders; and that the tumultuous and visibly spasmodic passions of joy and anger are all at least for a time maniacal. But these passions constringe the muscles of the head and neck, and therefore like a ligature force the blood that was descending in the jugular veins back upon the minutest vessels of the brain.

Spasm therefore, when it is productive of tumors by Fluxion or of sudden distensions in the vessels contiguous to the nervous substance, as also spasmodic passions such as joy and anger are to be reckoned amongst the remoter causes of Madness. Not but that the same muscular constriction is often excited by the application of several external objects; which objects are therefore to be added to the same class. For besides the many well attested cases of poisons or medicines, which as soon as swallowed convulse the body and intoxicate the understanding, such as Hemloc, and the root lately mistaken for Gentian, such as Opium when administered to some particular patients, &c. The many bottle-companions whose pulses beat high and quick, whose faces are flushed with blood in the same manner as if they were strangled, who are first wild and then stupid, who drink till they see double, and then drink on till they cannot see at all, as well

as

as the crowds of wretches that infest our streets and fill our hospitals, evidently prove to the vulgar as well as to the Physician that vinous spirits instantaneously provoke an irregular action of the muscles succeeded by temporary delirium; and that, if the same noxious draughts are taken in too large doses or frequently repeated, they become a very common tho' remoter cause of continual madness.

If any one rather supposes that such external objects, which produce Madness, act immediately upon the nerves thereby affected, and that spasm, tho' an undoubted effect of the same objects, is the companion and not the intervening cause of their delirious effect: However probable the contrary opinion may still appear to those, who consider that spasm never fails to precede or to accompany the nervous disorders subsequent to such application, and moreover that spasm is sufficient to produce maniacal symptoms; nevertheless the nearest known cause of Madness remains exactly the same, and these external objects are still to be reckoned among its remoter causes, which ever opinion is the more probable. Since it is impossible for any one of them to act at all upon the nerves without motion impulse and pressure in the same manner and order, as if they had previously occasioned muscular constriction

striction and vascular obstruction its most usual effect.

As for Tumors by Congestion ending in Madness, that is to say those loads of fluids which gradually overcharge the vessels contiguous to the nerves, and by compressing a sufficient quantity of medullary matter create delusive sensation as effectually as does inflammation or any sudden distension of the same vessels: such gradual or chronical congestions are frequently, tho' not always, an effect of a very different sort of muscular constriction, easily distinguishable from the former by its manner of invasion and continuance. For this spasmodic action of the muscular fibres is very gentle at first, and so far from alarming either the patient or his friends, that for some time it is very little attended to or even discernable. But what it wants in violence is more than made up by its obstinate duration and encrease: inasmuch as it seldom remits, and is with great difficulty relieved by art. This species therefore of spasm must likewise be added to the remoter causes of Consequential Madness.

To such constant muscular constriction, and to the gradual or chronical congestions in the brain or mesenteric viscera thereby occasioned, the

the despairing bigot, incapable in his own apprehension of being pardoned by infinite mercy, or predestined by infinite justice to eternal misery before he had a being, the moping lover, the motionless widow or mother bereft of her children, may at first view be ascribed. Who all wear *contractæ seria frontis*, and discover the fixed muscular marks of passions slower indeed in their operation than the turbulent storms of joy or anger, but which in consequence of pressure upon the nerves are as much the remoter causes of Madness, and indeed sooner or later are as destructive to every animal power.

The same Tumors by Congestion, capable with intervening pressure of creating Consequential Madness, are indeed oftentimes an effect of laxity in the overloaded vessels themselves. But even this weakness, if traced to its original, will frequently be found owing to one of the two aforementioned species of muscular constriction.

To such vascular laxity arising from muscular spasm may be referred the many instances of Madness occasioned by præmature, excessive, or unnatural Venery, by Gonorhœas ill cured with loads of Mercury and irritating Salts, by fevers, and other such like convulsive tumults. And from hence we may account for the chimærical dreams

dreams of infirm and shattered Philosophers, who after having spent many days and nights without closing their eyes in unwearied endeavours to reconcile metaphysical contradictions, to square the circle, to discover the Longitude or grand Secret, have at last fallen half asleep, and who by excessive attention of body have strained every animal fibre, and may without a metaphor be said to have cracked their brains.

But, altho' laxity arising from spasm is most commonly the cause of gradual obstructions ending in delusive Sensation, nevertheless the same delirious tumors by Congestion, more especially those that act upon the nervous matter contained in the abdomen, are formed sometimes without laxity or any spasmodic disorder whatever, either by excess of eating or by defect of voluntary motion: which motion is just as necessary to a due propulsion of the fluids thro' the uterine and hæmorrhoidal vessels, and thro' the many and intricate ramifications of the *vena portæ*, as is the action of the heart or the resilition of the vessels themselves. Gluttony therefore and idleness are both to be added to the remoter causes of Consequential Madness.

To the first is owing the meagrim of the Epicure. To the second, perhaps more than to a spirit of lying, may be afcribed the temptations of St. *Anthony* and the lazy Monks his followers, the extafies of fendentary and chlorotic Nuns, and their frequent converfations with Angelic minifters of grace. Not to mention what now and then happens to the fenior Reclufes in our Proteftant Monafteries at *Oxford* and *Cambridge*.

SECT.

SECT. IX.

The Diagnostic Signs of Original and Consequential Madness; and the Prognostic arising therefrom.

HAVING in the two preceding Sections discovered most of the causes of Madness that deserve our attention, and thereby divided this disorder into two species, viz. *Original* and *Consequential*: It will be necessary to mention some particular circumstances attending either species, which will enable the Physician not only to distinguish Original Madness from Consequential, but also the better to settle his prognostic and method of cure.

First then, there is some reason to fear that Madness is Original, when it neither follows nor accompanies any accident, which may justly be deemed its external and remoter cause.

Secondly, there is more reason to fear that, whenever this disorder is hæreditary, it is Original. For, altho' even in such case it may now and then be excited by some external and known cause, yet the striking oddities that characterise whole families derived from Lunatic anceſtors, and the frequent breaking forth of real Madneſs in the offspring of ſuch illconcerted alliances, and that from little or no provocation, ſtrongly intimate that the nerves or inſtruments of Senſation in ſuch perſons are not originally formed perfect and like the nerves of other men.

Thirdly, we may with the greateſt degree of probability affirm that Madneſs is Original, when it both ceaſes and appears afreſh without any aſſignable cauſe. For, although we cannot gueſs why this diſeaſe of the nerves is ever relieved without the real aſſiſtance of art, or why it attacks the patient again without any new provocation, any more than we can account for the ſpontaneous intermiſſion of convulſion, fever, head-ach, and ſuch like ſpaſmodic diſorders of the muſcles; it is however impoſſible that any one effect whatever can perfectly ceaſe, ſo long as that cauſe which was capable of producing it continues to act upon the ſame ſubject and in the ſame manner. And it is as impoſſible that the effect of any action can after a total diſcontinuance ariſe again, without its being regenerated by the ſame or at leaſt by a ſimilar action. Therefore that diſorder, be it muſcular or nervous, be it convulſion or Madneſs, which ſpontaneouſly ceaſes and as ſpontaneouſly invades again,

again, cannot be confequential to any external caufe, which always exifts, and whofe action always continueth the fame.

Original Madnefs, whether it be hæreditary or intermitting, is not removable by any method, which the fcience of Phyfick in its prefent imperfect ftate is able to fuggeft.

But, altho' Original Madnefs is never radically cured by human art, its illconditioned fate is however a little recompenfed fometimes by a perfect recovery, fometimes by long intervals of fanity, without our affiftance and beyond our expectation. Befides Original Madnefs is in itfelf very little prejudicial to animal life. For it is notorious that men, really mad live as long as thofe who are perfectly in their fenfes; and, whenever they ficken or die, they like other mortals are moft frequently attacked by illneffes, which have no neceffary connection with or dependance upon their old complaint of falfe perception.

Madnefs, which is confequential to other diforders or external caufes, altho' it now and then admits of relief by the removal or correction of fuch diforders or caufes; yet in proportion to the force and continued action of fuch caufes, and according

according to the circumſtances of the preceding diſorders, it is very often complicated with many other ill effects of thoſe cauſes and diſorders; and, tho' it may not in itſelf be prejudicial to bodily health, any more than Original Madneſs, yet by its companions it becomes fatal or greatly detrimental to animal life.

Madneſs, tho' it may be Conſequential at firſt, frequently becomes habitual and in effect the very ſame as Madneſs ſtrictly Original. In which caſe the internal frame and conſtitution of the nervous ſubſtance retains that ill diſpoſition which was communicated to it *ab extra*, even after that the cauſe of ſuch communication is quite removed or ceaſes to act: And the ſame ſubſtance, tho' formed originally as perfect as that of other men, yet by the continual and forcible action of ſuch external cauſe is at laſt eſſentially vitiated in the ſame manner and to as great a degree, as if it had been created imperfect and of itſelf capable of exciting deluſive ſenſation.

When internal exoſtoſes of the cranium, or induration of the Dura Mater are the cauſes of Conſequential Madneſs, each of theſe caſes is apparently incurable by art. Fracture or intropreſſion of the cranium, and concuſſion of the head, or rather its effects, tho' very dangerous and

and difficult to be managed, have sometimes been relieved.

When Insolation by the intervening rarefaction of the blood contained in the brain produces delirium, this its mischievous effect frequently yields to the lancet, if not too late or too sparingly applied. But if Madness is the more immediate consequence of the Sun's action upon the nervous substance, and if, however occasioned it is from want of care or from obstinacy of the case protracted after that the piercing darts of heat its remoter cause are quite abated, it is generally of long duration and very often incurable: forasmuch as the medullary portion of the brain is either shocked by the continued distension of the contiguous vessels, or is distracted by the fiery impression in such a manner that its constituent particles are quite deranged from that order, which is necessary to the performing their natural functions in a proper manner.

Madness consequential to the inflammation of those membranes that surround the brain is very dangerous: because such obstruction is formed in minute vessels which lie out of our reach, and which cannot be soon enough relieved by the most plentiful evacuation; nor can the brain thus overcharged endure any additional shock of errhines,

errhines, vomits, or rough purges: Since spasm thereby excited would either endanger a rupture of the distended vessels, or heighten the delirious pressure up to Apoplexy, or convert the inflammatory matter into mortification.

And indeed this state of Madness, called Phrenzy, let the Physician act ever so skilfully, frequently ends in one or other of the two last mentioned cases. The first of which is plainly threatened by stupidity succeeding to delirium; and mortification of the brain may be declared coming on, or rather formed, when the maniacal symptoms cease without any apparent reason, and when the patient who was raving becomes calm and sensible in an instant; whilst greater debility and a pulse hardly perceivable, together with coldness in the extremities, foretell that this unexpected recovery of the understanding, however it may flatter, will be fatal.

Madness consequential to a gradual or chronical congestion of fluids frequently admits of releif, if applied in time. And such congestion is less dangerous and more easily removed whenever the mesenteric nerves alone are thereby affected; inasmuch as every difficulty and danger that attends any injury must be less the fewer those nerves are that suffer the same.

When

When spasm is productive of obstructions upon the brain and nerves, and in this case becomes another and a still remoter cause of Consequential Madness, if such spasm is suddenly excited either by the tumultuous passions of joy and anger, or by intoxicating drugs and vinous spirits, it is indeed very violent and oftentimes fatal by its immediate effects. But in case the patient is capable of bearing the first shock, and has not been weakened by frequent attacks of the same nature; such sudden and irregular action of the muscles together with all its phrenetic or maniacal consequences is much sooner either spontaneously abated or relieved by art, than the gradual and continued muscular constriction, which is occasioned by the more gentle passions of love grief and despair, or by long and uninterrupted attention to any one object however pleasing and agreeable. For Madness consequential to such obstinate muscular constriction must be as obstinate as its cause: and besides in this case of continual or increased congestion, there is great reason to fear least the internal frame of the nervous substance itself may at last be essentially vitiated; and Madness which is habitual or of the same nature with that which is Original may succeed, and take the place of what at first was only Consequential.

Laxity, whenever it intervenes between fpafm and delirious preffure and thereby becomes a remoter caufe of Confequential Madnefs, admits of cure if timely and properly applied; and very often the weakened membranes fpontaneoufly recover their former elaftic tone, provided the fpafmodic impulfe is abated, before their conftituent fibres are diftracted beyond that natural tendency to approximation which was originally implanted in them.

Madnefs confequential to gradual or chronical congeftions occafioned by gluttony or idlenefs eafily yields to medical care, if feafonably and properly applied.

Madnefs confequential to or accompanied with other diforders affords no particular prognoftic, but what arifes from thofe diforders when confidered as primary diftempers diftinct and feparate from Madnefs itfelf.

Anxiety, when it arifes from fome fault inhæring in the internal frame and conftitution of the nervous fubftance, which is thereby rendered too fenfible, like Original Madnefs and for the fame reafon is not radically curable. But when its only caufe is a laxity or defect of thofe external

nal integuments which were given to the nervous fubftance for its defence, in fuch cafe Anxiety however afflicting promifes better fuccefs.

Infenfibility or Ideotifm, when it arifes from an internal and conftitutional defect of the organs defigned to excite fenfation, or when it is a fymptom or confequence of Original Madnefs, like Original Madnefs and for the fame reafon muft be pronounced incurable by art. But, what is very remarkable and much to be lamented, when Infenfibility is the effect of Confequential Madnefs, or when it may be attributed to the præternatural clofenefs and rigidity of the nervous integuments, or to obftructions in the contiguous veffels; tho' it may feem as curable as Confequential Anxiety, yet in fact (whatever is the reafon of the difference) it is very feldom relieved either by art or Nature.

SECT. X.

The Regimen and Cure of Madness.

THE Regimen in this is perhaps of more importance than in any distemper. It was the saying of a very eminent practitioner in such cases *that management did much more than medicine*; and repeated experience has convinced me that confinement alone is oftentimes sufficient, but always so necessary, that without it every method hitherto devised for the cure of Madness would be ineffectual.

Madness then, considered as delusive Sensation unconnected with any other symptom, requires the patient's being removed from all objects that act forcibly upon the nerves, and excite too lively a perception of things, more especially from such objects as are the known causes of his disorder; for the same reason as rest is recommended to bodies fatigued, and the not attempting to walk when the ancles are strained.

The visits therefore of affecting friends as well as enemies, and the impertinent curiosity of those, who think it pastime to converse with Madmen

and

and to play upon their passions, ought strictly to be forbidden.

On the same account the place of confinement should be at some distance from home: and, let him be where he will, none of his own servants should be suffered to wait upon him. For all persons, whom he may think he hath his accustomed right to command, if they disobey his extravagant orders will probably ruffle him to the highest pitch of fury, or if they comply will suffer him to continue in a distracted and irresolute state of mind, and will leave him to the mercy of various passions, any one of which when unrestrained is oftentimes more than sufficient to hurry a sober man out of his senses.

Every unruly appetite must be checked, every fixed imagination must if possible be diverted. The patient's body and place of residence is carefully to be kept clean: the air he breaths should be dry and free from noisom steams: his food easy of digestion and simple, neither spirituous, nor high seasoned and full of poignancy: his amusements not too engaging nor too long continued, but rendered more agreeable by a well timed variety. Lastly his employment should be about such things as are rather indifferent, and which approach the nearest to an intermediate

diate state (if such there be) between pleasure and anxiety.

As to the cure of Madness, this like the cure of any other disease consists, 1. In removing or correcting its causes: 2. In removing or correcting its symptoms: 3. In preventing, removing, or correcting its ill effects.

These three intentions are to be answered either by general and rational science; or, if that is wanting, by particular experience alone collected from plain and similar facts, which the history of practice supplies us with.

Original Madness indeed deserves our first attention, as it is the least complicated with any other disorder. But a very little reflection will serve to convince that all our consideration will never enable us to treat this first species of Madness in a rational manner. For it is impossible by any thing like judgment or previous design to answer the first intention, *viz. to remove the immediate necessary and sufficient cause of Madness*, which cause lies out of the reach even of our imagination: And, since no quality whatever can be corrected but by its contrary quality, therefore the unknown state of the nervous substance, when exciting delusive sensation, prevents our

our applying to it any remedy, whose apparent qualities betray a manifest contrariety to such distempered state.

And as to the second and third intentions, they in Original Madness are as little to be answered as the first. But that is not because either the symptoms or the ill effects of Original Madness lye out of our reach, or their causes are unknown; but because Original Madness when considered *per se* is not accompanied with any symptoms or succeeded by any effects, which if not prevented removed or corrected would endanger the life or health of the patient.

Nor does experience, which oftentimes supplies the defect of rational intention in many disorders that are hitherto inexplicable by general science and the common laws of Nature, furnish us with any well attested remedy for Original Madness. For, altho' several specifick Medicines have by the merciful direction of Providence been of late successfully applied in some distempers otherwise incurable by art, such as Mercury in the Venereal infection, Opium in pain and watchfulness, the Peruvian Bark in mortification intermittent fevers and many other complaints; and altho' we may have reason to hope that the peculiar antidote of Madness is reserved in Nature's ture's store, and will be brought to light in its appointed time; yet such is our present misfortune, that either this important secret hath been by its inventors withheld from the rest of mankind, or, which is more probable, hath never yet been discovered.

Since therefore the first species of Madness is incurable by any remedy which reason or experience suggests, let us divert our attention to the second species: And here to our great comfort we shall find that Consequential Madness is frequently manageable by human art.

For, altho' delusive Sensation, by whatever external accident it may be occasioned, when considered as a distempered state of the nerves themselves, admits of no rational or specific relief any more than Madness which is not consequential to any known cause; nevertheless the previous disorders and external causes of delusive Sensation are frequently within our reach. And this, as well as any other morbid effect, may in reason be and in fact often is prevented or abated; provided the known cause is taken care of in time, that is before its continued action hath altered the nervous substance to such a degree as to have rendered it essentially or habitually unsound.

Now,

Now, forasmuch as pressure of the nervous or medullary substance amongst all the known and external causes of Consequential Madness appears the nearest to its delirious effect, and indeed so necessary a cause, that without its intervention nothing external can be supposed capable of exciting delusive Sensation, this cause therefore must be the first object of our care.

In the next place our endeavours are to be employed in preventing removing or weakning those other external accidents before enumerated, which by occasioning intermediate pressure are the remoter causes of Consequential Madness.

Delirious pressure of the brain or medullary substance contained in the nerves, which is the nearest of all the known causes of Madness and therefore demands our first attention, is incapable of being effectually relieved, except the compressing matter itself be lessened, diverted, or dislodged from the part affected: or, to speak technically, the chief intentions under this first article are 1. Depletion; 2. Revulsion; 3. Removal; 4. Expulsion.

Not that all these intentions are to be answered in all cases and circumstances of delirious pressure.

pressure. For when internal exostoses, induration of the Dura Mater, fracture intropression and concussion of the head occasion such pressure, Removal (which indeed intropression does now and then admit) is apparently impracticable. Nor can Expulsion in any one of these cases, or indeed in any oppression of the brain that is similar to tumor by Fluxion, be attempted without imminent danger to the patient's life.

But the two first intentions are almost always to be pursued; and delirious pressure of the brain or medullary substance contained in the nerves demand Depletion and Revulsion, let its remoter causes or circumstances be what they will. For, tho' neither of these intentions propose the removal of exostoses or any one accident just now mentioned, yet unloading the vessels contiguous to the brain or nerves, which are thereby aggrieved, will certainly in all cases prevent or lessen the delirious effect. And, if the pressure arises solely from the distension of the vessels themselves, Depletion and Revulsion are apparently the apposite and necessary methods of relief.

When pressure of the brain or nerves is sudden, both these intentions may safely and effectually be answered by the lancet and cupping-glass again and again repeated in proportion to the strength of the patient and the greatneſs of the preſſure ; by neutral ſalts, which gently ſtimulating the inteſtines and ſenſible parts contained in the abdomen provoke ſtools and urine : of this ſort are Nitre, Sal Catharticus amarus, Magneſia alba, Tartar, and all its preparations, more eſpecially the Sal Diureticus deſervedly recommended by Dr. *Mead* in Maniacal caſes. And Revulſion in particular may be ſucceſsfully attempted by the oily and penetrating ſteams ariſing from ſkins and other ſoft parts of animals newly ſlain, by tepid fomentations and cataplaſms applied to the head legs and feet, by oily and emollient glyſters ; which are of very great ſervice not only as they empty the belly, but alſo and indeed chiefly becauſe they ſerve as a fomentation to the inteſtinal tube, and by relaxing the branches of the aorta deſcendens, which are here diſtributed in great number, make it more capable of receiving the blood; which will therefore according to the known courſe of fluid matter be diverted from the head.

The ſame intentions of Depletion and Revulſion ſeem indeed to recommend ſinapiſms, cauſtics, errhines, and veſicatories, as alſo the rougher cathartics, emetics, and volatile diaphoretics. But when we reflect that a ſpaſmodic conſtriction is by no means the leaſt amongſt the remoter

remoter causes of Madness, we shall in every case of sudden pressure be fearful of any powerful irritation that endangers constriction, and that cannot answer either intention unless it previously excites an irregular action of the muscles.

And indeed Phrensy or sudden pressure of the brain attended with inflammation of the containing membranes, and intrusion of blood and serum into improper vessels of the head, not only forbid sinapisms and every powerful irritation, but incline us to be suspicious of cathartic salts in too large doses, and even of Nitre itself, tho' it is reckoned specifically antiphlogistic, and tho' it is successfully administered in many other inflammatory tumors before they suppurate.

Delirious Pressure of the nervous substance contained either in the head or abdomen, when gradual or chronical, tho' it is of a very different nature from sudden pressure, and tho' it is similar to tumor by Congestion, yet in robust and plethoric habits alike indicates Depletion and Revulsion. But, if the subject is either naturally infirm or shattered and exhausted by preceding illness, the lancet must be cautiously used or entirely forbidden; and both these intentions can with safety be answered by nothing except the mildest solutives, such as the neutral salts abovementioned,

mentioned, Caſſia, Manna, &c. and the Gumms quickened with a few grains of Aloes.

But, when delirious preſſure of the nervous ſubſtance, more particularly that contained in the abdomen, is gradual or chronical, if ſuch gentle evacuants, tho' often and properly repeated, prove unable to leſſen or relieve the ſtagnating matter, and in caſe the weakneſs of the patient does not contraindicate, here the third and fourth intentions take place: and it becomes abſolutely neceſſary to ſhake with violence the head and hypochondria by convulſing the muſcular fibres with emetics rougher purges and errhines. For ſuch ſpaſmodic action communicates a vibrating motion to the ſolid fibres of the whole body; whereby the overloaded membranes and integuments that compreſs the contiguous medullary ſubſtance remove or expell their morbid contents, and the patient delivered from his delirious incumbrances frequently recovers his former ſanity of mind as well as body.

SECT.

SECT. XI.

The Cure of Madness.

PRessure of the medullary matter contained in the brain and nerves, amongst all the known causes of Madness the nearest to such its delirious effect, and therefore the first object of our attention, has been considered with regard to such methods of cure as are indicated by reason and justifyed by experience. In the next place therefore we are to turn our thoughts to those *other external accidents, which by occasioning intermediate pressure are the remoter causes of Consequential Madness.*

Now the several remoter causes before enumerated, were 1. Internal exostoses of the cranium; 2. Induration of the Dura Mater; 3. Fracture or intropression of the skull and concussion of the head; 4. Insolation; 5. One species of spasm, or muscular constriction, sudden and impetuous but sooner quieted; which arises either from 6. Material objects external to the body, *viz.* poisons, medicines, and vinous spirits, or from 7. Tumultuous passions, *viz.* joy and anger; 8. Another species of spasm or muscular con-

constriction more gradual and gentle in its attack, but frequently encreasing, and almost always obstinate in its duration; which arises from 9. Unwearied attention of the mind to one object, or from the quieter passions of love, grief, or despair; 10. Præternatural laxity of the membranes or vessels contiguous to the nerves; 11. Gluttony; 12. Idleness. Of all which in their order.

Internal exostoses and induration of the Dura Mater cannot be prevented, nor does either case admit of any particular method of relief. *Concussion* may itself indeed be sometimes prevented, but its ill effects can never be prevented or removed by any intention except that of Depletion and Revulsion recommended under the first article of cure. In *fracture or intropression of the skull* the trepan is peculiarly adapted either to give a vent to, or to remove the extravasated and stagnating fluids.

Insolation is quite out of our power; but its subject we have to deal with is not always so. For, altho' the fiery darts of heat are not capable of being removed or lessened by human means, the patient may be removed; or, when that cannot easily be done, the head may be secured by a proper integument; for which purpose a cap of of thick paper has been succesfully recommended.

Spasm or muscular constriction, as well the sudden and impetuous as the more gradual and gentle, when considered by its self and as abstracted from irritation or any external cause, admits of no method of cure suggested by rational intention: Forasmuch as the immediate necessary and sufficient cause of muscular action, be it natural or distempered, is absolutely unknown. Whenever therefore nothing external to the muscular fibres can be assigned which is capable of provoking their constriction, we have no hope except in specific remedies, that is in such drugs, whose antispasmodic virtues experience alone has discovered.

Under this head of antispasmodics every one, I suppose, will readily place Valerian, Castor, the Gumms, and Musk; and, were I at liberty to indulge a suspicion which has for some time occurred, I should be inclined to add Nitre, the Magnesia, the Sal Diureticus, as also all alcaline substances incorporated with acids, all neutral salts, and all alexipharmacs or diaphoretics: whose sudden efficacy in appeasing the paroxysms of feverish disorders which are apparently spasmodic can be attributed to no other known power, but

but such as hath an immediate influence upon the animal fibres endued with motion. Not that any thing more than conjecture is hereby proposed; which is to be admitted or not, as the conclusions of others arising from their own just reasoning and experience shall determine.

But, whatever class the virtues of Nitre and neutral salts &c. shall hereafter be ranked under, it may at present with great truth be asserted from observations already made that they are the only specific helps, which can be depended on with any probability of success or even with safety in fits of Madness attended with fury and violent spasmodic motions. And it is as certain that those other anti-spasmodic drugs which are poinant and irritating, *viz.* Valerian, Castor, and the gumms, are serviceable and indeed harmless only in the second or gradual and gentler species of muscular constriction.

Which observations by the way not only serve to distinguish what specific remedies are proper for either case of spasmodic Madness; but moreover suggest a caution to the Physician in the administring even Nitre and other saline febrifuges in spasmodic disorders whether delirious or not: because such sharp bodies when over-dosed or when applied to subjects too susceptible of irritation

tion may sometimes aggravate every symptom they are intended to relieve, and may become as mischievous as those other more poinant antispasmodics have frequently proved, when prescribed in all convulsive cases under the general and improper title of *Nervous Medicines*.

The same caution is likewise highly necessary when spasm is occasioned by the sixth class of remoter causes, *viz. poisons, medicines, vinous spirits*, or any assignable matter which actually excites an irregular motion of the muscles. For it is almost self-evident that in such case all additional irritation must increase every convulsive effect, and that even the most gentle saline remedies will be hazardous or at best inefficacious, until the material cause of spasm if superficial is removed by chirurgical assistance, if it be in the stomach or intestines until it is discharged by the force of vomits or purges, or if such means of expulsion be thought too violent until the offending matter is sufficiently enervated by diluting and absorbing medicines, or in case of extream necessity until its effect is prevented or stifled by narcotics. All which different methods of cure in such Consequential Madness must be left to the sagacity of the Physician; it being impossible to lay down any general direction in a

matter

matter attended with so great a variety of unforeseen accidents.

But, though the removal of the sixth class of remoter causes, *viz.* every irritation which produces Madness, is not always feasible or even safe, and though such terrible effect admits of no relief so long as the material cause continues to act, nevertheless prevention, at least with regard to vinous spirits, is entirely in our power. For which reason it deserves the serious consideration of our governors, how far it is their duty by a total prohibition of the cause to prevent those frequent effects of temporary but real Lunacy, for which many wretches are executed, who in reality are guilty of debauchery alone, which has been rendered familiar by the custom or rather the convenience of their country, and is allowed or commuted for by the laws of the revenue.

As to the seventh class of remoter causes, *viz. tumultuous and spasmodic passions, such as joy and anger*, in case the patient is not in immediate danger of his life, nothing of any great consequence is to be done at first; in hopes that these passions and their muscular effects will, as they are frequently known to do, subside of themselves. But, whenever *anceps remedium* is the indication, after sufficient depletion and diminution of maniacal preffure thereby occafioned, we muft have recourfe to the fpecific, that is to the unaccountably narcotic virtues of the Poppy. And, if notwithftanding this temporary relief any one particular paffion feems to engrofs the man or continues beyond its ufual period, in fuch cafe the difcretion of the Phyfician muft determine how far it may be advifeable or fafe to ftifle it by a contrary paffion. I fay *fafe*, becaufe it is almoft impoffible by general reafoning to foretell what will be the effect of fear fubftituted in the room of anger, or of forrow immediately fucceeding to joy.

The eighth remoter caufe of Confequential Madnefs, *viz. Mufcular Conftriction, gradual, gentler and uniform, but more obftinate*, may fometimes be relieved or as it were diverted by convulfion that is by an alternate motion of mufcular fibres artificially excited in fome other part of the body. On which account veficatories, vomits, rough cathartics, errhines, and the moft poinant amongft the medicines called nervous, may in this particular cafe of fpafm become even antifpafmodic. For, ignorant as we are and perhaps fhall always be of the reafon, experience has fhewn that, although many parts of the body may be convulfed together, one fpecies of fpafm however

however occasioned seldom fails to put an end to that other which before subsisted.

When the ninth class of remoter causes demands our care, *viz. unwearied attention to any one object*, as also *love, grief, and despair*; any of these affections will sometimes be annihilated by the tumultuous but less dangerous and sooner subsiding passions of anger or joy. But, if such instantaneous alteration from one extreme to the other appears either not feasible or too shocking to be attempted with safety; bodily pain may be excited to as good a purpose and without any the least danger. It being a known observation, though as much out of the reach of human reason as are most others which occur in the animal œconomy, that no two different perceptions can subsist at the same time any more than the two different species of morbid muscular action, *viz. the convulsive and the constrictive*. Therefore vesicatories, caustics, vomits, rough cathartics, and errhines, may be and in fact often are as serviceable in this case of fixed nervous Sensation as in obstinate muscular constriction, inasmuch as they all relieve and divert the mind from its delirious attention, or from the bewitching passions of love, grief, and despair.

The

The tenth remoter cause of Consequential Madness, *viz. Laxity* of those vessels or membranes that are contiguous to the nervous substance, apparently indicates such remedies as have the experienced though unaccountable efficacy of contracting the material particles which constitute an animal body. Of this nature is iron, vitriol, and mineral waters impregnated therewith: but above all, when nothing contraindicates, the bathing in cold or rather sea-water.

As to the eleventh and twelfth remoter causes, *viz. Gluttony* and *Idleness,* little is requisite for their particular cure: since, after proper evacuations, temperance is undoubtedly the apposite remedy of the one, and bodily exercise of the other. Both which means of present recovery and of prevention for the future may be effectually prescribed to men of either character, at least whilst they are actually mad and properly confined. For the diet of the glutton in such case is absolutely in the Physician's power. And, although it would be no easy task to perswade or even to force any person, whether a Lunatic or not, who has long indulged in idleness, to put his body in motion; nevertheless this state of inactivity may be artificially broke through by vomits, rough cathartics, errhines, or any other irritating

irritating medicines: which in this cafe therefore anfwer more than one intention, and not only difcharge or diflodge the delirious load of ftagnating fluids, but alfo by their convulfive influence upon the mufcles of the abdomen and indeed upon every animal fibre of the agitated body crowd as it were a great deal of exercife into a fmall portion of time, and that without the confent of the patient, or even the trouble of contradicting his lazy inclinations.

SECT.

SECT. XII.

The cure of the symptoms and consequences of Madness. And some observations upon the whole.

IT may be recollected that the cure of Madness, as well as of all other distempers, consists in 1. Removing or correcting its causes: 2. Removing or correcting its symptoms: 3. Preventing, removing, or correcting its ill effects.

A method of answering the first intention has been proposed in the two foregoing Sections: the symptoms and ill effects of Madness should therefore be our next care.

But Original Madness, as hath been before observed, is not necessarily accompanied with any symptoms or succeeded by any effects, that are strictly speaking insalubrious.

And indeed, with respect to Consequential Madness, whatever may accompany it as a symptom or follow it as a seeming effect, every such accidental disorder hath in reality no necessary connection with Madness itself: but is either resolveable

solveable into other injuries quite foreign to Maniacal affections; or, if it is owing to any one remoter cause of Madness, it is still no more than another effect of the same cause; which effect is just as capable of being thereby generated, whether Madness is or is not produced together with such symptom or before such consequence.

For which reason every symptom and every seeming ill effect of Madness, whether Original or Consequential, must be considered either as a primary distemper, or as the effect of some primary distemper, to which a proper method of cure is applicable separate and independent of Madness; and therefore it is not the subject of our present enquiry.

But, as Anxiety frequently precedes Madness like its cause or accompanies it like its symptom, and as Insensibility sometimes succeeds Madness like its effect; tho' both these præternatural states of Sensation are as distinguishable and actually separate from delusive sensation, as any other animal distemper is or can well be: the same reasons however, which required a more particular enquiry into the nature and origin of these two nervous affections, will excuse our endeavouring to investigate what method of cure the discovery

discovery of their causes may seem to indicate with any the least probability of success.

Anxiety then is either Original or Consequential. For, as hath been before observed, it may arise, 1. From some ill-conditioned state of the internal and proper substance of the nerves affected; 2. From the intolerable impulse of external objects, or from some defect in those integuments and membranes that surround the medullary matter, and when they are perfect defend it even from the natural action of bodies which would otherwise excite too lively a sensation.

Anxiety, when it is Original, resembles Original Madness, and for the same reason seems as much out of the reach of medical assistance: But in fact its case is more fortunate; and, tho' Original Anxiety is just as incapable as Original Madness of being relieved by rational intention, it is however frequently palliated by more than one specific remedy.

For wine, and even vinous spirits which are rightly forbidden to persons in perfect health, when occasionally administered as medicines to animal bodies agonising with exquisite sensation, beguile the distresses of mortals, and oftentimes procure

procure them tranquillity and happiness, to which they have long been strangers. And, altho' neither wine nor vinous spirits are adviseable in the vexatious symptom of watchfulness, which frequently attends upon Anxiety, whether accompanied by Madness or not; forasmuch as such poinant stimuli must irritate before their narcotic virtues can take effect; yet I have often prescribed the *Extractum Thebaicum* from one to five grains without any ill consequence to such mad patients as were uneasy and raving all the night as well as day. And, where extream weakness or some approaches to stupor rendered this powerful narcotic not quite so safe, Camphire and Sagapenum have afforded the same anodyne and soporific virtues, tho' not to so great a degree.

Nor ought any one to reject such temporary expedients, as unworthy the attention of a Physician in Original Anxiety, even tho' it should prove incurable by art; who considers that it is his duty to protract the misery of his fellow-creatures, if it be but for a moment; and that anodynes are absolutely necessary in every case of Consequential Anxiety, untill either the intolerable impulse of external objects can be entirely removed or weakened by such methods as particular circumstances require, or untill the nervous integuments can be restored to their natural firmness by the astringent virtues of the Peruvian Bark, iron, vitriol, mineral waters, and cold bathing; which are the proper and oftentimes effectual remedies, whenever Anxiety arises from the laxity or defect of those membranes that surround and defend the medullary matter.

Insensibility, Idiotism, Folly, or whatever name it is usually known by, is, as hath been observed, almost always beyond the power of rational or specific relief. Nevertheless, that nothing may be left untried, it seems adviseable to make general evacuations, and to contrive partial but constant discharges of the fluids from the head and neck by perpetual blisters, setons, and issues. It may likewise be of some service, if nothing contraindicates, to shake the whole solid frame by vomits, cathartics, errhines, and all sorts of tolerable irritation. To which may be added, but not without great caution, the subtle and penetrating particles contained in mineral waters drank at the fountain-head, and the concussive force of the cold-bath or sea-water.

But if Insensibility is constitutional, or owing to the firm and healthy structure of those solid membranes

membranes which sheath the nervous matter, such natural defect or impediment is incurable by art. However this state of stupidity may, at least by those who are endued with too lively a sensation, be deemed a kind of negative happiness, and rather to be envied than lamented.

And thus ends our inquiry into the causes effects and cure of Madness. But, before we quit this subject, it may not be improper to subjoin a few remarks, which will readily occur to every one who recollects the premisses, and is moreover satisfied of their reasonableness.

We have therefore, as Men, the pleasure to find that Madness is, contrary to the opinion of some unthinking persons, as manageable as many other distempers, which are equally dreadful and obstinate, and yet are not looked upon as incurable: and that such unhappy objects ought by no means to be abandoned, much less shut up in loathsome prisons as criminals or nusances to the society.

We are likewise, as Physicians, taught a very useful lesson, *viz.* That, altho' Madness is frequently

quently taken for one species of disorder, nevertheless, when thoroughly examined, it discovers as much variety with respect to its causes and circumstances as any distemper whatever. Madness therefore, like most other morbid cases, rejects all general methods, *v. g.* bleeding, blisters, caustics, rough cathartics, the gumms and fætid antihysterics, opium, mineral waters, cold bathing, and vomits.

For bleeding, tho' apparently serviceable and necessary in inflammation of the brain, in rarefaction of the fluids, or a plethoric habit of body, is however no more the adequate and constant cure of Madness, than it is of fever. Nor is the lancet, when applied to a feeble and convulsed Lunatic, less destructive than a sword.

And, altho' blisters, caustics, and sharp purges quickned with white Hellebore, and indeed all painful applications, not only evacuate and thereby relieve delirious pressure, but also rouse and exercise the body, and seem more peculiarly adapted to Insensibility when it is a symptom or consequence of Madness; nevertheless these and all pungent substances are to be tried with great caution, or rather are not to be tried at all in fits of fury. Nor does even defect of sensation allow their use, whenever such defect is

occasioned

occasioned by the preceding excess of the nervous energy, or when it is accompanied with spasm. As to black Hellebore, it is either not the drug which was recommended by the Antients and made *Anticyra* famous, or else it did not really deserve such recommendation. For after several trials I have not the least reason to think it of any service in Madness.

For the same reason the gumms and all fœtid antihysterics, which are undoubtedly serviceable in Madness arising from or complicated with some sorts of spasmodic disorders, are by no means even safe in all præternatural actions of the muscles: much less can such irritating objects be proper in that particular case of Madness which is attended with feaverish heat, which happens in a plethoric habit of body, or which follows an inflammatory obstruction in the brain.

As to Opium, notwithstanding what hath been before said concerning the great relief obtained by this powerful drug in some particular circumstances, it is no more a specific in Madness than it is in the Small Pox. For no good whatever can be expected but from its narcotic virtue, and much harm may arise therefrom when improperly administered. For it is almost self-evident that in Madness attended with debility

bility and languor, or which approaches towards stupor and insensibility, every thing that deadens sensation must be highly detrimental when given in a sufficient quantity, and may prove fatal when overdosed.

Mineral waters drank at the fountain head and bathing in the sea or cold fresh water have been sometimes chiefly if not solely relied on in the cure of Madness, more especially when attended with Anxiety and known by the name of Melancholy. Nevertheless such methods of relief are all apparently contraindicated, whenever there is sufficient reason to suspect that irresoluble congestions of the fluids clog the membranes contiguous to the nervous substance, or that the solids are strained beyond the possibility of recovering their natural elasticity. For in case of irresoluble congestions every drop of water, whether mineral or not, taken into the circulation will be added to the obstructing matter; and the contracting force of cold or of sea-water applied externally will make the same matter more incapable, if possible, of being resolved. And, when the solids are irrecoverably strained, they will be in great danger of rupture or at least of a farther disunion of their constituent particles by the expansive force of mineral springs, as well as by the rude shock of cold or of sea-water, which

which is very sensibly felt even by those bodies, whose solids are strong enough to bear the same without being hurt thereby.

Lastly with respect to Vomits, tho' it may seem almost hæretical to impeach their antimaniacal virtues; yet, when we reflect that the good effects which can be rationally proposed from such shocking operations are all nevertheless the consequences of a morbid convulsion, these active medicines are apparently contraindicated, whenever there is reason to suspect that the vessels of the brain or nervous integuments are so much clogged or strained as to endanger a rupture or further disunion, instead of a deliverance from their oppressive loads. The same objection equally holds good against such muscular irritation, whenever the vessels are contracted with excessive cold, or when their contents are rarefied by heat, as also in constitutions that are lax and feeble or naturally spasmodic, and in several other circumstances which need no particular description.

Besides, since the characters that distinguish Original from Consequential Madness are not always so clear and certain as to leave no room for error, and since Original Madness is not curable by any method which human reason or experience

perience hath hitherto been able to discover; we should take great care not to do harm where it is not in our power to do any good, and not dwell too long on endeavouring to remove the causes of Madness, which perhaps are only imaginary, more especially if the methods to be made use of are by no means indifferent. For which reason, whenever upon sufficient tryal not only of vomits but even of rougher purges, tho' rationally indicated at first, the patient grows worse or at least gains no ground, they are all entirely to be laid aside. For, if in any case the *juvantia* and *lædentia* supply us with medical knowledge, they most signally do so in disorders, whose nature we are not thoroughly acquainted with, and where reasoning *a priori* cannot certainly foretell the success of any one application.

Nor let us immediately despair at being obliged to withhold that assistance which seemed the most effectual, or conclude that, because the patient cannot be relieved by art, he therefore cannot be relieved at all. For Madness, like several other animal distempers, oftentimes ceases spontaneously, that is without our being able to assign a sufficient reason; and many a Lunatic, who by the repetition of vomits and other convulsive stimuli would have been strained into
downright

downright Idiotifm, has when given over as incurable recovered his underftanding.

To which remarks arifing as juft conclufions from reafoning upon the unavoidable action of vomits and rougher purges, I fhall beg leave to add fome cautions, which experience has fuggefted as neceffary to be communicated to the young practitioner, even when fuch active medicines are proper. *viz.* 1. If the feafon of the year is in the choice of the Phyfician, to prefer the Spring or Autumn, as being in neither extream of cold or heat : 2. Not to perfift in their ufe at any one time for a longer term than fix or eight weeks : 3. Even during that term to give a refpite every other or at leaft every third week from all drugs except the gumms, neutral falts, or gentle folutives : 4. As foon as the patient vifibly approaches to a ftate of fanity, entirely to difcontinue thefe and all other violent methods; that the animal fibres, which have been ftrained either by the caufes of Madnefs or perhaps by the means of removing them, may be at liberty to recover their natural firmnefs and juft approximation of particles, which a repeated concuffion will certainly prevent.

F I N I S.

REMARKS
ON
DR BATTIE'S
Treatise on Madness,

BY

JOHN MONRO, *M.D.*

Fellow of the College of Physicians, *London*;
AND
Physician to *Bethlem-Hospital*.

O Major, tandem parcas, Insane, minori.
Horat. Lib. ii. Sermon. 3.

LONDON:
Printed for JOHN CLARKE, under the *Royal-Exchange*.
MDCCLVIII.

ADVERTISEMENT.

MADNESS is a distemper of such a nature, that very little of real use can be said concerning it; the immediate causes will for ever disappoint our search, and the cure of that disorder depends on *management* as much as *medicine*. My own inclination would never have led me to appear in print; but it was thought necessary for me, in my situation, to say something in answer to the undeserved censures, which Dr. Battie has thrown upon my predecessors.

ERRATA.

Page 1. line 9. has given us — *dele* us.
    2. line 25. *for* though *read* if.
    8. line 17. *for* Anaschar *read* Alnaschar.
    Ibid. line 24. *for* ſtruk *read* ſtruck.
    12. line 19. *for* may *read* muſt.

SECTION I.

Of the definition of Madness.

AS I do not agree with the author of the *Treatise on Madness* in his first position, that this distemper is as * *little understood as any that ever afflicted mankind,* so neither can I assent to the reasons he has assigned for the † *defect of our knowledge* in this matter.

Aretæus, one of the most ancient writers in physick, has given us a description of this disease, in terms precise and elegant. We find in him an exact account of all the various symptoms, that are commonly observed in the different stages of it; indeed *Aretæus,* and other authors of antiquity, have, like some of the moderns, supposed causes that never existed; this foible excepted, they are by no means to be contemned; for they thoroughly understood the nature of this disorder, however defective they may have been in the management of it.

The first reason given for this defect of our knowledge is, that the ‡ *care of lunaticks has*

* p. 1.   † p. 2.   ‡ ibid.

been entrusted to empiricks, or at best to a few select physicians, most of whom thought it adviseable to keep the cases, as well as the patients, to themselves. Let the quacks be answerable for their own conduct; but in favour of the *select physicians* I can safely affirm, that they kept their patients to themselves, in no other sense than as the gentlemen of the faculty usually do, excepting, that the nature of this distemper, and the interest of the patient, require particular caution and reserve.

By the *few select Physicians*, I presume are intended the Physicians of *Bethlem Hospital*, whom I consider it as a duty incumbent on me, to defend against any injurious reflections. Those within our remembrance were men no less remarkable for their honour and integrity, than distinguished by their skill and experience in their profession; they did not discover any marks of that selfish disposition, imputed to them, or *thought it adviseable* to keep the publick in ignorance for their own private advantage. They made use of no mean arts, either to procure patients, or to keep them. And though the nature of their business required secrecy, yet their method of practice was open and publick; they freely gave their opinion, whenever applied for, either at a
con-

consultation or in writing. Nor did they ever pretend to any particular nostrum, or make use of * *antimonial vomits, strong purges, and hellebore*, as SPECIFICALLY *antimaniacal*. Though they did not publish their thoughts on a distemper which was more immediately the object of their care, that was not owing to any design of keeping their manner of practice a secret, but that they thought it disingenuous, to perplex mankind, with points that must for ever remain dark, intricate, and uncertain.

The second reason given for the *defect of our knowledge*, is the want of a † *precise definition*.

The author's definition of madness, as well as I can collect it, is this; ‡ *the perception of objects not really existing, or not really corresponding to the senses, is a certain sign of madness*; therefore DELUDED IMAGINATION *precisely discriminates this, from all other animal disorders*.

Definitions are of no use, unless they convey precise and determinate ideas; and if this be one of the right kind, I am very unfortunate in not being able to comprehend it. It is certain the *imagination* may be *deluded* where there is not the least suspicion of madness, as

* p. 2.   † p. 3.   ‡ p. 4, and 5.

by

by drunkenneſs, or by hypochondriacal and hyſterical affections; there may be real madneſs where the *imagination* is not affected; ſo that a *deluded imagination* is not in my opinion the true criterion of madneſs. The *judgment* is as much or more concerned than the imagination, and I ſhould rather define madneſs to be a *vitiated judgment*, though I cannot take upon me to ſay that even this definition is abſolute and perfect.

Aretæus in his deſcription of madneſs has the following remarkable ſentence; * "οἱδε μὲν γὰρ παραισθάνονται, κ̀ τὰ μὴ παρέοντα ὁρέυσι δῆθεν ὡς παρέοντα, κ̀ τὰ μὴ Φαινόμενα ἄλλῳ κατ' ὄψιν ἰνδάλλεται· οἱ δὲ μαινόμενοι ὁρέυσι μόνως ὡς χρὴ ὁρῆν, ὐ γιγνώσκυσι δὲ περὶ αὐτέων ὡς χρὴ γιγνώσκειν." *Theſe men (the melancholy) are miſtaken in their perception, they ſee objects that are not preſent, as if they were preſent, and they fancy they ſee what appears to no other perſon: whereas, thoſe who are furious, ſee exactly as they ought, but do not judge of objects as they ought to judge. That is, they ſee right, but judge wrong.* This obſervation, though not univerſally true, may very properly be applied to the manner in which madmen are frequently affected; and is ſo far

* *Aret.* p. 38. edit. *Oxon.* per *Wigan.*

of use, as to shew, that even the antients observed more faculties of the mind to be vitiated than one. Indeed this is sufficiently proved by the terms made use of by writers of different nations. *Tully* in his * *Tusculan* disputations remarks, that the *Greek* language wanted words to denote the peculiar differences of this disease, in which point he thinks the *Latin* tongue superior to the *Greek*, distinguishing between *insania* and *furor*, the last of which he calls *mentis ad omnia cæcitas*. Other writers have termed it *mentis alienatio*. The *French*, though they apply the words *foû* and *folie* indiscriminately to madness and folly, have yet many expressions extremely proper, and descriptive of this distemper, *alienation, derangement d'esprit, perdre l'esprit, perdre la raison, perdre le jugement*; from whence we may fairly conclude, that the abovementioned *definition*, which attributes the whole of this disease to any one faculty of the mind, taking no notice of the rest, is by no means a true *definition*.

From the observations I have had the opportunity of making on this distemper, I am pretty certain, there is no case in which the *judgment* is not vitiated; there are many, in

* Lib. 3.

which

which both *that* and the *imagination* are visibly hurt; some, in which the first is affected, and the last, as far as we can determine by appearances, untouched.

Can we say the *imagination* is more *particularly* affected or deluded, where not only *that*, but every other quality, which distinguishes a man from a brute, except a few unconnected incohærent words, seems totally obliterated? When we see a man for months (I may say years) together, not suffering even a rag of cloaths on him, lying in straw; and without shewing any signs of discontent, or attempting to do mischief, maintain an inviolable silence against all the applications of persuasion and force; what reason have we for calling this a *deluded imagination?* Those who have been so happy as to recover from this state, describe it no otherwise than a total suspension of every rational faculty. Their recovery seems like the awaking from a profound sleep, having seldom any recollection, or at least a very confused one of what has passed during their illness.

There is besides these another species of madness, of a very dangerous kind, in which the *imagination* does not seem to be any way concerned.

High

High spirits as they are generally termed are the first symptom of this kind of disorder; these excite a man to take a larger quantity of wine than usual, (for those who have fallen under my observation in this particular, have been naturally very sober) and the person thus affected, from being abstemious, reserved, and modest, shall become quite the contrary; drink freely, talk boldly, obscenely, swear, sit up till midnight, sleep little, rise suddenly from bed, go out a hunting, return again immediately, set all his servants to work, and employ five times the number that is necessary; in short, every thing he says or does, betrays the most violent agitation of mind, which it is not in his power to correct; and yet in the midst of all this hurry he will not misplace one word, or give the least reason for any one to think he *imagines* things to exist, that really do not, or that they appear to him different from what they do to other people: they who see him but seldom, admire his vivacity, are pleased with his sallies of wit, and the sagacity of his remarks; nay his own family are with difficulty persuaded to take proper care of him, until it becomes absolutely necessary from the apparent ruin of his health and fortune. Nobody can doubt that this is real

real madness, and yet it is giving a very unsatisfactory account of the thing, to call it a *deluded imagination.*

Though I should allow the *imagination* to be the seat of the distemper, it would not follow that a DELUDED *imagination* is the proper definition, because it concludes too much; by taking in every delirium arising from fever, or from other causes: the truth of which is exemplified in the story of * *Alnaschar* ; however, ludicrous it may seem to produce it on this occasion, it is nevertheless a strong proof in support of what I have advanced; for the author in this story has with great good sense as well as humour given us a lively picture of a DELUDED *imagination,* without the least suspicion of insanity. Anaschar *had laid out all he was worth in glasses which he was to sell again, with the money which these goods will bring, says he, I shall purchase jewels, and at length, become a rich merchant, marry the visir's daughter, but am resolved to keep her in proper subjection; having said this, upon the first exertion of power, he struk the glasses down with his foot, and put an end to all his visionary expectations.*

* Vid. Spectator, No. 535.

Before

Before I leave this subject, I cannot help expressing my surprize, that a gentleman so ready to censure the inaccurate manner in which the generality of mankind express their thoughts, should be so careless in a matter that requires the greatest precision. In one paragraph madness is called a * *deluded imagination*, in the next † *false perception*, and *perception* is either confounded with, or not sufficiently distinguished from *sensation*; yet I cannot think these three the same; for how close soever the connection may be between *sensation* and *perception*, there is certainly a very wide difference between either of them and *imagination*.

SECTION II.

Of the seat, the supposed and real causes, and the salutary effects of natural sensation.

THE *seat, causes* and *effects* of *natural sensation*, take up no less than four sections of the *treatise*. There would not be the least objection to an *investigation of this kind*,

* P. 5.   † P. 6.

could it be done in such a manner as to advance our knowledge: but if after all, we can discover nothing more than that the medullary substance is the *seat*, and the nerves are the instruments of *sensation*, I can see no benefit that is likely to arise from it. Whether *sensation* itself is owing to pressure, or whether pressure is only the remoter cause, and there may be still required a * *different juxtaposition of the medullary particles previous to the immediate cause*, is a point I shall very readily submit to be settled by those who are inclined to † *fight in earnest with shadows*.

Nor am I any way desirous of entering into a dispute whether the nerves are tubes containing a fluid, or solid fibres acted upon by various causes; but as the question is by no means so far settled, as this author would insinuate, I should not look upon it as a ‡ *solemn confutation of chimæras* only, should any one endeavour to produce good reasons in favour of the solidity of the nerves; neither on the other hand, should I think those, who have maintained a contrary opinion, deserve the severe censure of *insanity*; as many of them have approved themselves expert anatomists, good physicians, and great philosophers.

* P. 25.   † P. 16.   ‡ Ibid.

While

While this point remains so undetermined, it is no wonder if we should sometimes be guilty of * *inaccuracy*, when we are speaking of the nerves, or the diseases which do, or seem to affect them.

Weakness of nerves, whatever objection is made to it, is a common phrase, and conveys to us a known idea, without leading us to consider whether it † implies, that *sensation itself is owing to the loose cohæsion of the material particles which constitute the nervous substance*, or not. And notwithstanding the great ‡ *danger of blending the most distinguishing property of animal nature with inanimate matter*, I am very much afraid we must still make use of it, until some more exact author than has hitherto appeared, shall supply us with a better. Though I will not take upon me to defend the accuracy of this expression, I see no reason why this gentleman should be so offended at it, who has not scrupled throughout his work to use the § *ill-conditioned state of the nerve*, ‖ the *disuniting and breaking in pieces of the nervous substance*, it's §§ *imperfection*, and *degeneration*, as if they were terms perfectly un-

* P. 17.   † Ibid.   ‡ Ibid.
§ P. 34.   ‖ P. 38.   §§ Ibid.

derstood, and to which mankind had affixed certain ideas.

We have now got over this *enchanted ground*, and are coming to the *real* causes of natural *sensation*, which however * *perplexed to the too curious enquirer,* are † *clear in idea to the modest observer, and fully to be accounted for, at least to all useful intents and purposes, as any phænomenon whatever.* Although this may very possibly be the case, I would still advise the reader in his perusal of ‡ this section to pass over the § *seven considerations on causes*, and some other paragraphs, lest he should be reckoned to have more *curiosity* than *modesty*. Afterwards indeed we meet with nothing but what is extremely plain, and of which I believe few have doubted; ‖ we are informed that *before an external object can create any sensation whatever, it may produce several intermediate effects, viz. motion, impulse, and pressure.* ¶ *Pressure*, we are told, *cannot be imagined without some alteration in the former arrangement of those material particles which constitute the nervous substance,* and *⁎* farther than this we are not allowed to penetrate.

* P. 19.   † Ibid.   ‡ Sect. iv. of the treatise.
§ P. 21, and 22.   ‖ P. 24.   ¶ P. 25.
*⁎ P. 26.

The

The *seat of sensation*, the *supposed and real causes of it*, having afforded little amusement, and in my opinion as little real knowledge, I was in great hopes a relation of it's * *salutary effects* would make us some amends, as these are points of general concern, and in which every one has an interest; but even here I must own myself greatly disappointed; for I can discover nothing new and entertaining, except the ingenious manner in which these are accounted for; this I must confess is so striking, that I cannot pass it by without notice.

The first of these *salutary effects* is very common, and what I should have imagined every one to have been perfectly well skilled in, it being nothing more than *eating* and *drinking*, which it seems were intended for the relief of those † *agonizing sensations, hunger and thirst*. It is amazing what an advantage a man of learning has over the ignorant; for while the one ‡ *looks no farther than the actual pleasure which accompanies the stifling such sensations*, he who is § *skilled in the animal œconomy*, knows not only the efficient and coercive causes which torment him to such good purpose, but is at the same time fully satisfied, that they were designed ‖ *by the Author of nature for the*

* P. 27.   † P. 28.   ‡ P. 29.   § Ibid.   ‖ Ibid.

refection

refection of the human body; and perhaps it is from hence that physicians, who are supposed to be well skilled in the animal œconomy, have been generally esteemed connoisseurs in these articles; but the latter part of the paragraph informs us of a thing I should scarce have believed even of this degenerate age, which is, that there are some people so unaccountably idle, that were it not for * *hunger and thirst, they would not give themselves the trouble of opening their mouths, much less by hard labour earn food wherewith to fill them.*

Respiration, or the † *introduction of fresh air into the lungs*, is the next effect of *sensation*; this it seems is of equal advantage to both learned and unlearned, and performed by both with equal ease, and herein no man suffers by idleness, because he can by no means ‡ *omit* the performance of this necessary office let him be ever § so *careless* or *obstinate*.

As to the third, namely *exercise*, I shall not at all dispute it's being necessary for the preservation of health; but according to the peculiar sense in which the word *anxiety* is used throughout this section, it plainly carries this ridiculous meaning with it, that a man who eats and drinks with the best appetite, who

* P. 29.   † Ibid.   ‡ P. 30.   § Ibid.

enjoys

enjoys a free respiration, and uses all voluntary exercise of the body, is one of the most anxious uneasy mortals upon earth, of which his appetite, his respiration, and his frequent exercise are all strong signs.

SECTION III.

Of anxiety and insensibility.

AS the discovery of new diseases enlarges the province of the physician, the Faculty are under great obligations to the author of the *Treatise on Madness*, who has furnished them with no less than two in one * section.

The *anxiety* often observed in fevers and other disorders is very well known; but this cannot be what is here meant: I presume restlessness and inquietude, not uncommon symptoms at the beginning of madness, may be intended. How *anxiety* in any shape should be *mistaken* for madness is to me unaccountable, nor did I ever meet with such a notion but in † this treatise.

It is said to arise from ‡ *disordered, not deluded sensation*; this subtle distinction on so intricate a subject is not quite satisfactory, and I

* Sect. vi.   † P. 5.   ‡ P. 33.

could

could have wished we had been favoured with a more plain account of a distemper, which is said to be frequently attended with the * *fatal consequence* of *suicide*. It is not impossible but my ignorance in this point may arise from the little regard I have hitherto paid to metaphysical enquiries, in which I have generally observed much labour used to cover the want of real knowledge. In order therefore to be better informed, I have selected such passages as seem to stand most in need of being explained; these I have drawn out, and have some thoughts of proposing them as prize questions, (in imitation of the *French*) to the academicians of *Bethlem*, where it is among the *senior recluses* only that I can expect to find any one, who is able to resolve them all.

I. † *If the quantity of concomitant affection, is not proportionate and therefore not in all respects corresponding to the natural quantity of it's real cause, will it not have some deviation from absolute truth?*

II. ‡ *Is the ill-conditioned state of a nerve inhærent in the internal, proper and unknown constitution of the medullary substance? or is it from the defect, or loss of those membranes*

* P. 37.   † P. 34.   ‡ Ibid.

which

which envelope and sheathe the seat of sensation?

III. * *What is the common share of sensibility a nerve is endued with in a body cloathed with skin?*
IV. † *Will the sensation of the nervous or medullary fibres, though they continue the same, be in a reverse proportion to the cohæsion of those minute particles, which constitute the solid and elastick fibres?*
V. ‡ *Whether nerves, that are pillowed with fat, soaked in lymph, or stifled by obstructed vessels, can or do receive a proper, that is a sensible impulse from external objects forcibly and rightly applied, although the nervous substance itself is in it's internal constitution fitted for the efficacious reception of such external impulse?*

Notwithstanding these questions may be esteemed very curious, I cannot but think they come far short of the clear and accurate description given of these new distempers. One way, in which they are said to be produced, has something in it so extraordinary, and so very new in physick, it is at least upon

---

* P. 35.   † Ibid.   ‡ P. 39.

that account worthy our attention. * The STRAINING *or loosening the solid parts of human bodies frequently render those bodies liable to be violently affected*; which violent affection is *anxiety.* This † *anxiety* by STRAINING *the instruments of sensation may produce insensibility*; this last *strain* must undoubtedly be of great service, for we afterwards find that *insensibility* is a kind of ‡ *negative happiness*, *or a state rather to be envied than lamented, at least by those who are troubled with a too lively sensation,* that is *anxiety.*

I shall conclude this section, with the author's account of these distempers in his own words, as best capable of conveying his meaning.

That I may be fairly understood, I shall suppose myself, for example, to be troubled with this § *habitual disease of anxiety*, and instead of dispatching myself, determined first to consult a learned physician; to whom after having told my case, I will suppose myself to say; pray doctor what is the cause of this *anxiety?* why sir, ¶ *it may be owing to the too great or too long continued force of external objects,* ‖ *or to the ill-conditioned state of the nerve.*

* P. 36. † P. 38. ‡ P. 93. § P. 37.
¶ P. 34. ‖ Ibid.

2

This

* *This ill-conditioned state of the nerve may be inherent in the internal proper and unknown constitution of the medullary substance, or it may arise from the loss or defect of those membranes which sheathe the seat of sensation.* But † *whatever cause it is owing to, it chiefly discovers itself in an agonizing impatience observable* OF *black* November *days,* OF *easterly winds,* OF *heat, cold, damps,* &c. Dear doctor, I thank you, just my case; you have hit it exactly,—but after this agonizing impatience goes off, I am as it were in a kind of *insensibility,* from whence proceeds that? that sir, nothing easier to be accounted for; that ‡ *may proceed from the anxiety that preceded;* or § *from the too close texture of the fibres that compose those integuments which sheathe the nervous substance;* ‖ or it may be owing to *the internal unknown constitution of the substance itself;* but ** *whatever cause it is owing to, it's ill effects are very obvious.* It is easy for the reader to imagine, that this learned account of my physician, affords just as much satisfaction to my mind, as relief to my distemper.

* P. 34. † P. 36. ‡ P. 38. § P. 39. ‖ P. 38.
** P. 39.

SECTION IV.

Of the causes of Madness.

THAT part of the treatise which I propose to examine in this section, does *really* and truly treat of madness; where no doubt we shall meet with great perspicuity, and sound reasoning, nothing systematical, nothing built on idle theory or weak supposition, nothing but what is the result of diligent and faithful observation. Yet here, even here, alas! the *unknown cause* like the *Anima* or *Archæus* of other philosophers is still too prevalent; though I must confess it is in one instance at least introduced to good purpose, and were it brought in for no other reason than to account for *original madness*, it would be harmless enough.

Of what use it may hereafter prove to have thus divided madness into * *original* and *consequential* is not my business to enquire at present. The first of these is entirely the doctor's invention it never having been mentioned by any writer, or observed by any physician.

* P. 44.

What

What is the cauſe of *original* madneſs? it is unknown. What the ſymptoms? there are none. The method of cure? it admits of no cure, unleſs * *nature has a mind to recompence a little it's ill-conditioned fate by a perfect recovery without our aſſiſtance and beyond our expectation.*

However ſtrange this account of *original* madneſs may appear, I ſhould have been glad if the whole firſt ſection on *the cauſes* of madneſs had been as eaſy to be underſtood; for I cannot help ſaying, that far the greateſt part of it ſeems not to be the object of *vulgar apprehenſion*, though there is an attempt to explain it by ſome very familiar alluſions; the firſt of which, viz † *ſtriking a man on the eye*, it may be proper to mention, becauſe it is a proof of what I before advanced with regard to definition; for if a violent blow on the eye excites the ſame idea of fire in the imagination, as real fire would do, if it acted upon the ‡ *material particles of the medullary ſubſtance of the optick nerve in a man awake*, when the idea is referred to a wrong cauſe, the error does not lie in the *imagination*, but in the judgment.

If by an attempt to diſcover the cauſes of madneſs we were led to any thing, that in our

* P. 61.   † P. 42.   ‡ Ibid.

practice

practice might prove a relief to those who labour under this distemper, it would be well worth our utmost endeavours to succeed in it; nay though it were not attended with so great a blessing, yet it would be something to say in it's favour if it afforded the mind any thing that deserved the name of a rational amusement; but by all I have been able to make out of the three sections on the *causes* of this disease, I do not find we discover more of them than we did before of the cause of *sensation*; for *pressure*, we are told, excited sensation, and here it is said to excite madness.

In ascertaining the causes of *sensation* and *madness*, the consequence of a mistake in either is by no means the same; the first, being only a speculative point, though in the discussion of it we should lay too great a stress upon conjecture, yet all the inconvenience arising from thence, would be very inconsiderable: but in fixing the *causes of madness*, we ought to be extremely cautious not to admit any, but such as we have the greatest reason to believe are certainly true; because in this case our mistakes may prove detrimental, and even fatal; as this is therefore a point of some moment it will be necessary to consider it with greater exactness.

Whether

Whether *original* madness arises from an *
internal disorder of the nervous substance, is beneath all serious consideration; I shall therefore pass over this question; and proceed to the diagnostick signs, by which we are to distinguish this kind of madness, from *consequential*; and it is very observable that when we endeavour to point out the difference between them, *fear* operates more than *reason*.

I. † *There is some reason to* FEAR *that madness is original when it neither follows, nor accompanies any accident which may be justly deemed it's external and remoter cause.*

The reasons in general assigned for madness are so deceitful, that I believe we do not know the true cause of the distemper in one third of those unfortunate persons, who are intrusted to our care; we should not therefore rely too much on private opinion and conjecture; it sometimes approaches by very slow degrees, it takes it's rise, like many other diseases, from small beginnings; and though it is certain that the effect did immediately follow the cause, yet it's first attack having passed unnoticed it is no wonder, it should afterwards be referred to

* P. 43.   † P. 59.

a wrong cause, or be supposed not to have arisen from any. This is more generally the case when madness is said to have been caused by love or drink, which are much oftener the *effect* than the *cause* of it.

II. * *There is more reason to* FEAR *that, whenever this disorder is hereditary it is original.*

If *hereditary* madness be *original,* and we are allowed to judge from experience, we have no reason to apprehend that it is an incurable disorder; for *hereditary* complaints of this nature are as often treated with success, as when they arise from a *known cause.*

III. † *We may with the greatest degree of probability affirm, that it is original, when it both ceases and appears afresh without any assignable cause.*

This as well as the first reason may and most probably does arise from want of exact observation. Is it not strange that a disease should be thought less curable, because it has already been relieved by nature without the assistance of art? or, why is *madness* to be so

* P. 59.   † P. 60.

particularly distinguished from other distempers, many of which cease and appear again without our being able to assign the real cause? It is a complaint the most liable to a relapse even where the cause is known, and why may it not cease *spontaneously* without being stiled *original*, when we afterwards find that * *sudden spasm* where it is mentioned as the occasion of *consequential* madness, may *spontaneously abate with all it's maniacal consequences*?

I should never have taken so much notice of this chimerical distemper, had it not been for the terrible doom pronounced against it, *that it is not to be cured*; by which means it must often happen, that a person labouring under madness (should he chance to be attended by a philosophical physician) must be abandoned as an incurable for no other reason, but because it has pleased this gentleman to create a new distemper under the name of *original* madness.

Again, † *original madness is in itself very little prejudicial to animal life. For it is notorious that men really mad live as long as those who are perfectly in their senses; and whenever they sicken or die, they like other mortals are attacked by*

* P. 65.   † P. 61.

illneſſes that have no neceſſary connection with madneſs. It is very ſtrange that madneſs ſhould be thought little prejudicial to animal life, *becauſe* madmen are ſubject to other diſeaſes. That the generality of madmen are long lived, I take to be a vulgar error.

Although I do not remember to have ſeen more than four inſtances, where I could ſay the fury of madneſs was the immediate occaſion of death, I have great reaſon to believe that *madneſs* deſtroys two thirds of thoſe who are afflicted with it through life. They are very ſubject to apoplexies, and to ſtrong convulſions, which frequently end in death, beſides other chronical and lingering diſeaſes brought on by obſtinacy, the uſual unhappy companion of this diſorder; we may indeed find among them ſome inſtances of long life, but they are far from being ſo numerous, as to juſtifie our calling it a common caſe: it is the lot of thoſe only whoſe mental faculties ſeem to be totally obliterated, and who ſhew little or no attention to any thing that paſſes; this, joined to the regular manner in which they are obliged to live, will carry a ſtrong, healthy conſtitution to a great age; however theſe examples are not ſo common as is generally believed, but confined in a great meaſure

to

to those, who have a fortune sufficient to supply them with the best attendance.

Thus ends the history of *original* madness; and the difficulties that occur upon this subject must be ascribed either to the uncertainty, or to our total ignorance of it's real *cause*.

But we shall be embarrassed with no more inconveniencies of this kind, as we are now come to the consideration of *consequential* madness; for here we have no less than twelve *causes* to assist us, though like *Touchstone*'s in the play, they are all *causes removed*; however, such as they are, I shall beg leave to examine them, because *this* distemper is allowed to be curable by art.

1, 2. * *Internal exostoses of the cranium*, and an † *induration of the dura mater*, may possibly produce madness; but as they are cases that, I presume, seldom happen, and when they do are beyond our knowledge, and confessed to be out of our reach, it can be of no use to consider them.

3. If real madness, not a delirium, should be the consequence of a ‡ *fracture* or *intropression of the skull*, or of *concussion*, I am afraid, all attempts to relieve it would be vain. I

---

* P. 62.   † Ibid.   ‡ Ibid.

never saw an instance of the first, and shall therefore say nothing about it; the last indeed, I have had frequent opportunities of observing, but do not remember to have seen it cured.

4. Although it might be questioned whether * *insolation* be a proper term for what is here meant, I have no design to dispute it's propriety in this place; but it would be kind in the author to inform his reader, whether it be from *anatomy* or *conjecture*, that we are authorised to say, the † *constituent particles of the medullary portion of the brain are quite deranged from their natural order by this cause of madness*.

5, 6. Here I must take the liberty to change the order in which these causes stand, and defer the consideration of the six next, which depend upon *spasm*, until I have enquired into the two last, viz. ‡ *gluttony*, or the *excess of eating*, and § the *defect of voluntary motion* vulgarly called *idleness*.

These two vices are said to occasion madness; what another person affirms himself to have seen, I should pay some regard to; had this been the case in the instances before us, it would certainly have induced me to believe

* P. 63.   † Ibid.   ‡ P. 66.   § Ibid.

they

they might have had such an effect; but unless I see it myself, or have credible information of it from another, common prudence requires me to suspend my belief. *Inactivity* or *indolence* is one very common *effect* of madness, but I cannot think it ever to have been the *cause*; *gluttony* does certainly produce variety of distempers; but as I have seen innumerable cases of madness, and never yet met with one which was reported to have arisen from either *gluttony* or *idleness*, I must wait for more convincing proof, before I can readily admit them as certain *causes* of madness.

The nature of system is so bewitching, that when once a writer becomes enamoured of it, he seldom fails to make his reason subservient to his hypothesis.

The learned author of the treatise is so very sensible of this foible, and the mischief that may ensue from it in the practice of physick; that in most of his works he has very loudly and justly exclaimed against it: in that before us he has said that *Theorists deserve the suspicion of insanity*. I would therefore be cautious in advancing any thing, that might seem to imply he had unadvisedly been guilty of such an error himself; yet I cannot persuade

suade myself but that the doctrine of *spasm* is liable to great suspicion.

I do not think he has by any means clearly established it as a cause of madness; nor is it made more intelligible or less systematical, by the notion borrowed from writers in surgery, of *tumours by fluxion* and *tumours by congestion*.

If I rightly understand his meaning (which I am afraid is not always the case) he seems to admit * that spasm may of itself excite maniacal symptoms: if so why are these *tumours* introduced? † or if external objects can excite madness by immediate pressure upon the nerves, I see no reason for the introduction of spasm. He seems not insensible himself, of the difficulty that may attend his doctrine, for it is easy to observe he is not quite certain whether *spasm* may not be the ‡ *companion* rather than *the intervening cause of delirious pressure*; and indeed in the famous description of anxiety, it is reckoned as one of it's § *morbid effects:* notwithstanding all which, he concludes that the ‖ *nearest known cause is still the same*, that is *pressure*; though this may very possibly be true, yet there is certainly a great deal of difference, between considering spasm as the cause pro-

* P. 54. † Ibid. ‡ P. 54. § P. 37. ‖ P. 54.

ducing

ducing madneſs, or only as a ſymptom attendant upon it ; ſince we are in the cure directed to apply medicines to it as a *cauſe*.

It may poſſibly be one of the effects of madneſs, but I ſhall doubt of it as a *cauſe*, until I ſee much plainer proofs of it than I have yet been able to find.

7, 8, 9. *Spaſm* eſtabliſhed upon no better foundation than this is ſuppoſed to be the *cauſe* of madneſs, and as ſuch is diſtinguiſhed into two ſorts ; * one, *ſudden* and *impetuous*, occaſioned by *joy, anger, vinous ſpirits*, and *intoxicating drugs* ; three of theſe may certainly produce madneſs, but the fourth does not, for the *effect* of *intoxicating drugs* ought not to be looked upon as any thing more than a temporary delirium, and for this I have the authority of † *Aretæus*.

10, 11. The more *gradual* and continued ‡ *muſcular conſtriction*, we are informed, ariſes from *long and uninterrupted attention to one thing*, from *deſpair, grief*, and the *gentle paſſion of love* ; here I cannot help obſerving what ſeems to me another inſtance of the fondneſs for ſyſtem : *love*, when it is ſaid to produce *anxiety* only, is a § *turbulent paſſion* pro-

* P. 65.   † P. 37. edit. Oxon.   ‡ P. 65.
§ P. 37.

voking

voking *perpetual tempests*; but when it is introduced as the *cause* of the greater evil *madness*, the *turbulence* ceases, and it becomes * *a gentle quiet passion*.

12. Again, † *laxity* is introduced as *intervening between spasm* and *delirious pressure:* had it been said, that *laxity occasioned* this *pressure*, we might with some reason have looked upon it as one of the remoter *causes* of madness if it is occasioned by pressure, but as the *delirious pressure* must have existed before *laxity* could intervene, I do not see why it is to be ranked among the *causes*. I know very well that a total relaxation of the fibres, is one common effect of *melancholy*; but *laxity* as it is here mentioned, is as far above my conception as *spasm*.

I much wonder that, in the enumeration of the causes of madness, two of the most obvious should have escaped notice; sudden frights, and obstructions in women; the first hardly ever effectually cured, the last extremely difficult to be removed.

Should any one see this long list of *causes*, of which madness is said to be the *effect*, would he not imagine that each *cause* produced invariably or at least generally its parti-

* P. 65.   † P. 66.

cular

cular *effect?* more especially when he observes in the cure of this distemper, that peculiar medicines are adapted to each particular *class* of *causes*, would he not have reason to conclude that the madness arising from one, was of a different nature from that produced by another? or that joy and hatred occasioned a madness greatly different in its appearances from that which arose from grief and love? yet if any one depending upon this doctrine should think so, he would be miserably deluded in his imagination, and a little experience would soon convince him, that although the causes differ as much as is possible, the distemper is still the same; joy and hatred, love and grief, will occasion a madness attended with symptoms sometimes different, at other times exactly the same.

When drink is the *cause* of this disease, it shews less variation in it's *effect* than when it takes it's origin from any other cause; but this can only be said when it follows a sudden debauch; for if it happens after a long and continued course of drinking, there appears nothing particular, that will lead us to guess at the *cause*.

The immediate causes of madness are so very intricate, and so far beyond our comprehension,

hension, that we never can expect any satisfactory account of them. Am I better acquainted with *sensation*, for being told that *pressure* is the nearest known cause of it? Or, if I have not some notion of delirious pressure, am I likely to know more of madness, when I am informed it is the consequence of *delirious pressure?* Will the author venture to affirm that a passion of the mind, joy for example, does produce *madness* in the following manner? Joy occasions a sudden and impetuous *spasm*, this causes tumours by fluxion, and from thence proceeds *delirious pressure*, which is *madness*. Is this absolute truth, or only conjecture? If it be not truth, it can never be of any service, and may certainly tend to deceive us.

As an enquiry into matters so far out of our reach, cannot be attended with any real satisfaction, we may employ our time to much more advantage, than in such fruitless searches.

The effects of this distemper are plain and visible, let us therefore direct our knowledge to relieve *them*, and make use of such methods as are warranted by reason, and founded upon observation and experience; leaving the causes of this terrible calamity, which will for ever remain unknown, to such as can fancy there is any amusement in a disquisition of so unpleasing a nature.

SECTION V.

Of the regimen and cure of madness.

AS by *regimen* I presume is meant the *management* necessary for the cure of madness, I am thoroughly sensible, it is a point of the last importance, and in which the judgment and knowledge of the physician are of the utmost consequence.

If by the words * *eminent practitioner in such cases* the author means the late physician of *Bethlem*, the publick does not want to be informed, he was infinitely superior to such a news-paper compliment; to say he understood this distemper beyond any of his cotemporaries, is very little praise; the person who is most conversant in such cases, provided he has but common sense enough to avoid metaphysical subtleties, will be enabled by his extensive knowledge and experience to excel all those who have not the same opportunities of receiving information. He was a man of admirable discernment, and treated this disease with an address that will not soon be equalled. He knew very well, that the *management* requisite

* P. 68

for it was never to be learned, but from obfervation; he was honeſt and fincere, and though no man was ever more communicative, upon points of real uſe, he never thought of reading lectures, on a ſubject that can be underſtood no otherwiſe than by perſonal obſervation; phyſick he honoured as a *profeſſion*, but he defpiſed it as a *trade*; however partial I may be to his memory, his friends acknowledge this to be true, and his enemies will not venture to deny it.

Management is univerſally allowed to be of the greateſt moment, but other perſons befides the phyſician muſt be concerned in this part, though they are to act under his direction; it may therefore be expected, that what we meet with on this head will be ſuited to common capacities, that it may be rendered more uſeful to the publick in general.

Let us then obſerve the rules, that are laid down to direct us in this point.

* *People who are mad ſhould not be waited upon by their own ſervants, but confined at a diſtance from home, in a dry air, free from noiſome ſteams; where neither friends, nor enemies ſhould be allowed to viſit them, nor any one be ſuffered to play upon their paſſions; their unruly appetites*

* P. 68, and 69.

muſt

must be checked, their fixed imaginations diverted, their rooms and their perſons kept carefully clean; they ſhould have good plain victuals, not high ſeaſoned; their amuſements ſhould be various, and their employment indifferent.

In ſuch a manner is a doctrine of the higheſt conſequence in this diſtemper delivered, with a brevity, that would ſcarce afford matter enough for a lecture of five minutes; for even adorned with all the arts of circumlocution, ſo frequently to be met with in this performance, it ſtretches no farther than two pages, while the leſs important part of *medicine* takes up very near thirty.

Both reaſon and experience ſufficiently convince us of the neceſſity of *confining* ſuch as are deprived of their ſenſes; it is certainly of the utmoſt ſervice, and has reſtored many without the aſſiſtance of *medicine*; though I ſhould hardly think it ſafe to truſt to this alone.

Such confinement is more likely to be of ſervice abroad, than at home; and the country is preferable to the town for the opportunities it affords of uſing exerciſe, without the danger of being expoſed.

It is doubtleſs unreaſonable to appoint a ſervant to be his maſter's governor, nor are thoſe who are afflicted in this manner ever ſo well

or

or so easily managed as by strangers, over whom they have no authority. They should at first converse with few. Great art should be made use of in breaking all ill habits, and they should be checked, if their conversation runs too much on one subject. The physician should never deceive them in any thing, but more especially with regard to their distemper; for as they are generally conscious of it themselves, they acquire a kind of reverence for those who know it; and by letting them see, that he is thoroughly acquainted with their complaint, he may very often gain such an ascendant over them, that they will readily follow his directions. They should be accustomed to obey, and though talked to kindly, it should still be with authority. They should be used with the greatest tenderness and affection, nor, were it possible to prevent it, should their attendants ever be suffered to behave otherwise to them; when they do, they betray their trust; much less should they on any account endeavour to make them do what is required by frightening them, for though they may sometimes compass their ends by such means, it is never without danger, and has often added to the misery of the unhappy patient.

It

It is likewise a good general rule not to permit their friends to visit them, but would those, who intrust their relations to our care, put so much confidence in the physician, as to let him judge of the propriety, it need not be always rigorously observed; there are times, when such visits are highly detrimental, yet they may be sometimes permitted without any bad consequences, and I have frequently known them of service; but all this should be submitted to the judgment of the physician; who, if he has that honour and humanity he ought to have, will act as much like a friend as a physician in such deplorable cases.

I should scarce have thought it worth while, under this head, to have mentioned cleanliness as a necessary article, since nothing but the most gross and unpardonable negligence, can leave any one to suffer by the want of it, in this, or any other distemper.

Little is to be said with regard to diet, their meals should be moderate, but they should never be suffered to live too low, especially while they are under a course of physick; they should be obliged to observe great regularity in their hours; even their amusements should be such as are best suited to their disposition; but the employment here recommended

mended is certainly one of the moſt ingenious that was ever invented; it muſt be ſomething of * *an intermediate ſtate between pleaſure and anxiety.* Well indeed might the author add, *if ſuch there be.*

With regard to *management*, it is ſometimes of conſequence to know the *cauſe* of the diſorder; not ſo much to direct us in the choice of medicines, as in the manner of conducting ourſelves towards the patient: every one is not to be accoſted in the ſame manner, ſome are to be commanded, others are to be ſoothed into compliance, but we ſhould endeavour in every inſtance to gain their good opinion. It is impoſſible to be ſo full on this ſubject, as not to leave many things unſaid; much will depend upon the care and attention of the phyſician, whoſe method muſt vary according to the complaints of his patients; in this branch, neglect or ignorance will admit of no excuſe: and I am very ſure that *management* has not yet reached the perfection of which it is capable.

From theſe obſervations on *management* we might proceed to that of the cure of madneſs, in which *medicine* is concerned; if it were not

* P. 70.

for the new doctrine of *original* madness, which we are cautioned not to attempt the cure of as the *cause* of it lies beyond the * *reach even of our imagination*; nor should we endeavour to remove the † *symptoms* or *ill-effects* of it, though *they should lie within our reach*, *because they are not dangerous either to the life, or health of the patient*: indeed *experience*, however instructive in other cases, cannot furnish us with a *specifick* against a complaint, that never was heard of until this book was published; I am however glad to see the author is so sanguine in his expectations, that this *specifick is reserved* ‡ *in nature's store*, from whence, I hope, his deep researches may bring it forth to publick view, no person being so likely to find out the remedy as he who found out the disease.

Consequential madness, happily curable by art, though brought on by so many different *causes*, will not suffer from the want of *medicine*; for here every thing that goes under that name finds a place; but application must be made in time, before § *the nervous substance is altered to such a degree*, as to become *essentially and habitually unsound*; what is meant by the alteration of the nervous substance, to an *unsound*

* P. 70.   † P. 71.   ‡ P. 72.   § Ibid.

G   *state,*

state, is beyond my comprehension; it approaches so near to the unknown *cause*, that I wish this gentleman, who has before taken the pains to explain to us what ought to be meant by *weakness of nerves*, had condescended to fix such ideas to these expressions, as would have made them intelligible.

The cure of *consequential* madness is not inferior to the rest of the performance, containing many remarks very singular in their kind; the manner in which it's different species are ranged under their several *causes*, and the particular *medicines* adapted to each, would be of great use to us, and save an infinite deal of trouble were it possible to put it in practice; for by this method every thing would follow of course, when we were once made acquainted with what had been the *occasion* of the distemper.

1, 2. *Internal exostoses of the cranium*, or *an induration of the dura mater, cannot be prevented, nor does either case admit of relief.*

3. The * *trepan* we are informed is *peculiarly adapted to the removal of extravasated fluids*, when they are the consequence of a fracture. The † *ill effects of concussion are not easily prevented or removed, though concussion it-*

* P. 79. † Ibid.

self

self may be sometimes prevented; if this gentleman has any receipt for that purpose, it would be of such universal use, that it is not quite fair to keep it a secret; for it can scarce be imagined that he meant, it might be prevented by it's not happening.

4. * *Insolation, is quite out of our power, but it's subject we have to deal with is not always so*; the meaning here, though so strangely expressed, is nothing more than this; we cannot prevent the sun from shining, but we may sometimes remove a man out of it; or where that is not to be done, we may provide him *a proper integument*, i. e. a paper cap.

5. † *Spasm, when considered by itself and abstracted from irritation, or any external cause, admits of no method of cure suggested by rational intention.* This kind of *original spasm*, for it arises from no apparent cause, though abandoned by *rational intention,* is not to be given up as desperate; for we are in this case directed to apply to † *specifick remedies, whose anti-*

---

* Ibid. If it were worth while to criticise upon words, I do not think *insolation* is a proper term; for as far as I can trace it out it means nothing more either in Latin or English, than exposing to the sun: nor do I remember to have seen it used in either language to signify the effect the sun has upon bodies; this the Latins called *solatum,* and those affected by it *solati.*

† P. 80.   ‡ P. 80.

spasmodick

spasmodick virtues experience alone has *discovered*; and it will be very hard, if we do not meet with some among these, that will serve our purpose; for most of the *materia medica* seems to be comprehended under the title of *antispasmodick* in one part or other of this *treatise*.

6. The methods of cure proposed in the sixth class, being all of them uncertain, must be left to the * *sagacity of the physician*; one case only excepted, which is recommended to the † *serious consideration of our governors*; who are desired to think of some remedy to prevent *the temporary but real lunacy*, occasioned by the drinking of *vinous spirits*.

7. When madness succeeds *anger* or *sudden joy*, the cure, it seems, is readily found, if we can but once persuade ourselves, it will succeed; for we are ‡ *at first to do* NOTHING OF ANY GREAT CONSEQUENCE *if the patient be not in immediate danger of his life — in hopes these passions and their muscular effects will subside of themselves*; but if they should not, and § ANCEPS REMEDIUM *be indicated, after sufficient depletion and diminution of the maniacal pressure* THEREBY *occasioned, we are to have recourse to the unaccountably narcotick virtues of the poppy*. And if notwithstand-

* P. 82.   † P. 83.   ‡ Ibid.   § Ibid.

ing

ing these judicious applications the case should still prove obstinate, the physician is then to determine, * *how far it may be safe to substitute fear in the room of anger, or make sorrow succeed to joy.* The first, I am certain, is dangerous, and the last contradictory to common sense: a surgeon might as well pretend, that to break a man's arm was the most effectual cure for a broken leg.

The doctrine of substituting one passion for another is of very antient date, but I will never subscribe to the errors of antiquity, in opposition to experience, reason and common sense. It has indeed been known, that frights and passions of the mind suddenly excited, have produced very good effects in some cases; but we are not from thence to conclude, that they ought to be prescribed; for were the history of their good and bad effects fairly laid before us, we should see the balance greatly on the side of the latter. When one prevailing passion has already proved too powerful, and the mind, obstructed in it's operations, is become weaker from that cause, is it reasonable to suppose that it will be so well able to bear the shock, or receive any benefit from the attack of another? it certainly will not; and I should think

* P. 84.

there is reason to apprehend the most dangerous consequences from an abrupt and sudden alteration of the passions where we sometimes see the mind violently agitated from mere trifles.

8. The eighth *remoter* cause of madness is another kind of *spasm* which may be likewise stiled *original*. This contains nothing very remarkable, it is* *gradual, gentle, uniform, but more obstinate* than the first; and is to be *relieved* or *as it were diverted* by *convulsion artificially excited* by *means of vesicatories, rough catharticks and errhines.*

9. † *Unwearied attention of the mind to one object, love, grief, and despair*, are supposed to be sometimes the cause of this second species of *spasm*. Could an alteration of the passions be here effected by gentle degrees, we might more reasonably expect success from it than in the instances before-mentioned; but I have already said enough on that head. The other remedy proposed, I should little have expected to have seen prescribed by a physician: ‡ *bodily pain may be excited to good purpose, and without any the least danger.* Though *bodily pain* in general be here recommended, I presume that only is meant which arises from

* P. 84. † P. 85. ‡ Ibid.

medicinal

medicinal application: but can any man think of laying on * *blisters* and *causticks*, of giving *vomits* and *rough catharticks* with no other design than to excite pain? *Celsus*, and some other authors, mention *beating* as serviceable, but such kind of treatment is deservedly exploded at this time, as unnecessary, cruel, and pernicious. I never saw the least good effect of *blisters* in madness, unless it was at the beginning, while there was some degree of fever, or when they have been applied to particular symptoms accompanying this complaint.

10. † *Laxity*, one of the *remoter* but unaccountable *causes* of madness, may very well demand medicines of an *experienced, though unaccountable efficacy*.

11, 12. Little is requisite for the particular cure of madness when it is the consequence of ‡ *gluttony* or *idleness*; for, *after proper evacuations, temperance is undoubtedly the apposite remedy of the one, and bodily exercise of the other*: that is, gluttony is cured by being a glutton no longer, and idleness by being no longer idle. § These are the *means of present recovery, and of prevention for the future, which may be effectually prescribed to men of either character, at least while they are actually mad and properly confined.*

* P. 85.   † P. 86.   ‡ Ibid.   § Ibid.

But

But it seems to me a confused way of speaking, to talk of *prevention for the future*, while a man is in an *actual state of madness*.

The description * *of putting idleness in motion*, that is of making inactivity active, is entertaining, and may possibly to some people seem *philosophical*; *this state of inactivity may*, though not without difficulty, *be artificially broke through by irritating medicines, which will not only dislodge the delirious load of stagnating fluids, but also by their convulsive influence on the muscles of the abdomen, and indeed upon every animal fibre of the agitated body, croud, as it were, a great deal of exercise into a small portion of time.*

When I observed this gentleman at his first setting out representing madness, as a distemper *but little understood*, though several authors had professedly written upon the subject; and blaming others for not publishing their thoughts upon it; I was in hopes to have met with something new or useful in his own performance; either a more accurate description of the different appearances of the distemper, or at least something, that might lead us to a method of practice more advantageous to our unhappy patients. The manner indeed of ranging mad-

* P. 86.

ness under several *causes* is new, but will not, I fear, be of any great use.

The first *intention* in the cure of this distemper is the removal of it's *causes*; now out of twelve here set down, how many are to be removed by medicine according to the author's own doctrine? the first and second are given up by himself; little or nothing is recommended to be done in the third and fourth; the fifth is not to be cured by *rational intention*; the cure of the sixth is *uncertain*; and the seventh is to be relieved by *the narcotick virtues of the poppy*; the eighth to be diverted *by convulsion artificially excited by medicines adapted to that purpose*; the ninth by the same kind of medicines made use of to *excite bodily pain*; in the tenth we are directed to remedies of *an unaccountable efficacy*; the eleventh and twelfth are to be cured *by proper evacuations*. So that out of the twelve *causes*, there are hardly more than two, that are to be removed by *rational intention*; and it is a doubt with me, whether either of those two have been ever known to produce madness.

Upon the whole, I cannot help thinking, that this section has been expressly written, to prove the truth of what was asserted by the *eminent practitioner* at the beginning of the last,

last, viz. *that management did much more than medicine in this disease.*

Notwithstanding we are told in this *treatise*, that madness rejects all general methods, I will venture to say, that the most adequate and constant cure of it is by evacuation; which can alone be determined by the constitution of the patient and the judgment of the physician.

The evacuation by *vomiting* is infinitely preferable to any other, if repeated experience is to be depended on; and I should be very sorry to find any one frightened from the use of such an efficacious remedy by it's being called a * *shocking operation, the consequence of a morbid convulsion.* I never saw or heard of the bad effect of *vomits*, in my practice; nor can I suppose any mischief to happen, but from their being injudiciously administered; or when they are given too strong, or the person who orders them is too much *afraid of the lancet.*

The prodigious quantity of phlegm, with which those abound who are troubled with this complaint, is not to be got the better of but by repeated *vomits*; and we very often find, that *purges* have not their right effect, or do not operate to so good purpose, until the

* P. 97.

phlegm is broken and attenuated by frequent *emeticks*.

Why should we endeavour to give the world a shocking opinion of a remedy, that is not only safe, but greatly useful both in this and many other distempers? however, to obviate the apprehensions, that may be conceived from such an account, it would be worth while to peruse some cases related by * Dr. *Bryan Robinson*, who does not seem to have been at all alarmed at this *shocking operation*, which, he tells us, he has prescribed for a whole year together, sometimes once a day, sometimes twice, and that with the greatest success.

I lately received from a worthy friend of mine the case of a gentleman, who had laboured under a melancholy for three years; he himself calls it an hypochondriacal, convulsive disorder, from which he was relieved entirely by the use of *vomits*, and a proper regimen. So very sensible was he of their good effects, that he did not scruple to take sixty-one from the third of *October* to the second of *April* following; and for eighteen nights successively one each night; by which means he got rid of a prodigious quantity of

---

* Observations on the virtues and operations of medicines, p. 145. & seq.

phlegm, and obtained a perfect recovery. The firſt ſeventeen were compoſed of one ounce of the vin. ipecacoan. with one grain of emetic tartar, and afterwards he made uſe of no more than half an ounce of the wine. And thoſe, who are much uſed to hypochondriacal people, will find them in general leſs weakened with *vomits* than *purges*.

Bleeding and *purging* are both requiſite in the cure of madneſs; but *rough catharticks* are no otherwiſe particularly neceſſary in this diſtemper than on account of the phlegm, and to conquer the obſtinacy of the patients, who will ſometimes fruſtrate the operation of more gentle medicines.

Iſſues between the ſhoulders, have been often of great ſervice in the removal of this diſtemper; cold bathing likewiſe has in general an excellent effect, but as it is ſometimes apt to hurry the ſpirits, it is not to be preſcribed indiſcriminately to every one.

Alteratives are often, if not always neceſſary, and in moſt circumſtances may be employed to advantage. As to *the peculiar antidote of madneſs reſerved in nature's ſtore*, it will be ſoon enough to talk of *that*, when *it ſhall be brought to light in it's appointed time.*

SECTION VI.

Of the cure, of the symptoms, and consequences of madness. And some observations upon the whole.

THE cure of madness, as well as of all other distempers, consists in, I. the * *removing or correcting it's causes*; this has been already treated of in the foregoing section; there remain now to be considered the second and third *intentions* of cure, which are † II. *the removing or correcting it's symptoms*, and III. *the preventing, removing, or correcting it's ill effects.*

Here I expected to have met with a regular detail of the *symptoms* and *ill effects* of this distemper; but to my great astonishment, in the following paragraphs we are told, that there are *no bad symptoms* or *ill effects*, which ‡ *have in reality any necessary connection with madness itself.*

Without any aggravation therefore, we learn nothing more from these directions, but that madness is madness, which we are to cure by *removing* or *correcting it's causes*, though we cannot get at them; *by removing* or *correcting it's*

* P. 88. † Ibid. ‡ Ibid.

symptoms,

(54)

symptoms, though it has none; and by *preventing, removing,* or *correcting it's ill effects,* though it is followed by none that *in reality* belong to it.

The medical part of this performance is equally clear and improving; in one page we have the pleasure to see, * *that consequential madness is manageable by human art* ; in another we have the mortification to find, that the *characters,* which distinguish *original* madness from it, † *are not always so clear and certain as to leave no room for error.* ‡ In this doubtful state we are to be cautious of attempting a cure, *for fear of doing harm when it is not in our power to do any good;* though in another part of this work, we are advised to put in practice several methods in cases § *almost always beyond the power of rational or specifick relief, that nothing may be left untried.*

‖ *We are taught as physicians a very useful lesson* which no one ever doubted; that, although madness is frequently taken for one species of disorder, yet when thoroughly examined it discovers as much variety with respect to it's causes and circumstances as any distemper whatever.

* P. 72.   † P. 97.   ‡ P. 98.   § P. 92.
‖ P. 93, 94.

We

We are likewise taught, that * *like most other morbid cases, it rejects all general methods,* and if the methods explained by the v. g. † are to be called general methods, and applied without judgment or discretion, common sense will for once join with madness, and reject them too.

What man ever thought ‡ *bleeding the constant and adequate cure of madness?* § Who ever *relied on mineral waters as it's chief or sole remedy?*

|| *Black hellebore,* whether it be *the same drug recommended by the antients* or not, may be used to good purpose, though it is no *specifick:* but is it necessary, that physicians should be cautioned not to give *irritating medicines* ¶ *in madness attended with feverish heat?* *⁎* *in plethorick habits, or which follows an inflammatory obstruction in the brain?* are they solemnly to be told, that *⁑* *opium is no more a specifick in this distemper than in the small pox?* or may we not suppose them to have judgment and knowledge sufficient to find out these mighty matters without being thus directed?

* P. 94.   † P. 94, *bleeding, blisters, causticks, rough catharticks, the gums, and fœtid antihystericks, opium, mineral waters, cold bathing, vomits.*   ‡ Ibid.   § P. 96.
|| P. 95.   ¶ Ibid.   *⁎* Ibid.   *⁑* Ibid.

I

I declared myself of a different opinion from this gentleman at the beginning of these remarks, and have as little reason to agree with him now I am drawing towards the end of them, especially in his last conclusions.

* I. *If the season of the year is in the choice of the physician, to prefer the spring or autumn, as being in neither extream of cold or heat.*

This is supposing a case that never can exist; the season of the year is not in the choice of the physician; it is his duty to apply himself to the cure of his patient as soon as he is called in, not suffering the distemper to gain ground by waiting and wishing for more favourable weather; that the success of medicine in cases of this kind, does not depend upon the season of the year in which it is applied, is manifest from a recent instance: I never remember so many patients discharged well in any one year from *Bethlem* hospital, as were discharged thence last year, though the spring was cold, and the summer hot in an extraordinary degree.

† II. *Not to persist in the use of vomits and purges at any one time for a longer term than six or eight weeks.*

* P. 99.   † Ibid.

This

This is a very improper direction, and if strictly followed will be an effectual means of retarding the cure. When evacuations are not carried beyond the patient's strength, nor crouded too fast upon him, his health of body will visibly improve, by continuing them beyond the groundless and chimerical restriction of eight weeks.

As I think the second conclusion too cautious, I cannot help looking upon the third as trifling.

* III. *Even during that term* (six or eight weeks) *to give a respite every other or at least every third week from all drugs, except the gums, neutral salts, or gentle solutives.*

The meaning of these two paragraphs taken together amounts to this; you are not to put your patient into a course of *vomits* and *purges* for more than eight weeks at a time; and even during that time you must omit the *vomits* at least every third or every other week; these are contradictions which nobody but our author can reconcile.

† IV. *As soon as the patient visibly approaches to a state of sanity, entirely to discontinue these, and all other* VIOLENT METHODS.

I am at a loss to conceive what can be meant by *other violent methods*; but to prevent

* P. 99.   † Ibid.

a rea relapse, I am convinced, there is a necessity of continuing in some measure the regimen, even after the cure is compleated; and I shall strengthen what I have advanced with the words of Dr. *Mead*, where he closes the account he has given of this distemper. " * There is no disease, in which the danger " of a relapse is greater; wherefore every thing " that has been hitherto proposed for the cure, " whether relating to medicines, diet, or man-" ner of living, ought to be repeated for a " considerable time at due intervals, even after " the patient has recovered."

Had Dr. *Mead* been more conversant in this complaint, than he was, we might have expected greater improvements from him; but short as his observations are, they contain one very true and curious remark, which I do not remember to have seen in any other author; " that some dangerous distempers have " suddenly disappeared at the coming on of " madness "

To this I will add another observation, for which we are indebted to the last physician of *Bethlem*; that an intermitting fever coming upon a madness of long standing, the relief of that has proved the cure of the madness; of this I have seen two instances myself, and one

* Monita medica translated by *Stack*. p. 101.

of them in a man who had been extremely ill for three years.

The only cautions neceffary for thofe who are unacquainted with this complaint are; not to be too hafty in their evacuations, nor to carry them beyond the ftrength and conftitution of the patient: never to lofe a proper authority over him, which they will always find requifite for his management; not to be impofed upon by his cunning artifices; nor to give him up too foon as an incurable. As to medicines, there can be no particular directions; all that are proper in other diftempers, will be found of ufe in this, when applied with judgment.

Before I have done, it is impoffible to help taking notice of one thing, which has to me appeared very extraordinary on perufing this work; that of the many *fymptoms*, certainly and conftantly attending this diftemper, the author has not thought proper to beftow a fingle obfervation on any one. We are indeed told, they fhould be removed, but without fo much as being enumerated, they are made * *primary diftempers*, or *the effects of primary diftempers*, and are no more heard of. This feems to be great affectation of fingularity,

* P. 89.

and

and of so strange a kind, that I think every prudent writer should endeavour to avoid it; but especially, such as treat of physical subjects; for they will perpetually fall into mistakes about the disease, if they have not a particular attention to the symptoms: which very thing has happened in the book before us, where the author says, that Dover had the good luck to cure a * *Calenture by mistaking it for the plague*; what foundation he has for saying so, no man can imagine; if we believe the account given by Dover, there can be no doubt of the distemper; the symptoms enumerated, which are many, being certainly pestilential, and at the same time there is not one peculiar to the *Calenture*.

Having gone through the observations, that occurred to me upon this extraordinary performance, it must now be left to the impartiality of the publick to determine between the Treatise and the Remarks.

If Dr. Battie should have † *miscarried in his undertaking*, I cannot think that the *judicious reader will be* HEREBY *inclined to turn his thoughts to the same subject.*

* P. 47.   † P. 3.

F I N I S.